Gaucher Disease

AF670832

Parastoo Rostami • Ali Talea
Editors

Gaucher Disease

An Updated Guide to Diagnosis and Management and patients presentation

Springer

Editors
Parastoo Rostami
Research Center for Growth and Development, Division of Endocrinology and Metabolism, Department of Pediatrics, Pediatrics Center of Excellence
Tehran University of Medical Sciences
Tehran, Iran

Ali Talea
Metabolic Disorders Research Center, Molecular-Cellular Endocrinology and Metabolism Research Institute
Tehran University of Medical Sciences (TUMS)
Tehran, Iran

ISBN 978-981-96-4762-0 ISBN 978-981-96-4763-7 (eBook)
https://doi.org/10.1007/978-981-96-4763-7

© The Editor(s) (if applicable) and The Author(s), under exclusive license to Springer Nature Singapore Pte Ltd. 2025

This work is subject to copyright. All rights are solely and exclusively licensed by the Publisher, whether the whole or part of the material is concerned, specifically the rights of translation, reprinting, reuse of illustrations, recitation, broadcasting, reproduction on microfilms or in any other physical way, and transmission or information storage and retrieval, electronic adaptation, computer software, or by similar or dissimilar methodology now known or hereafter developed.
The use of general descriptive names, registered names, trademarks, service marks, etc. in this publication does not imply, even in the absence of a specific statement, that such names are exempt from the relevant protective laws and regulations and therefore free for general use.
The publisher, the authors and the editors are safe to assume that the advice and information in this book are believed to be true and accurate at the date of publication. Neither the publisher nor the authors or the editors give a warranty, expressed or implied, with respect to the material contained herein or for any errors or omissions that may have been made. The publisher remains neutral with regard to jurisdictional claims in published maps and institutional affiliations.

This Springer imprint is published by the registered company Springer Nature Singapore Pte Ltd.
The registered company address is: 152 Beach Road, #21-01/04 Gateway East, Singapore 189721, Singapore

If disposing of this product, please recycle the paper.

Preface

Inborn errors of metabolism (IEMs) are single gene disorders, which are rare in the whole world, but collectively, they are more common in some races and populations, especially in populations where family marriages are carried out. Increasing the awareness of pediatricians about these disorders is critical in the early diagnosis and treatment of these patients. Recent developments of newborn screening programs and availability of whole exome sequencing to confirm of diagnosis and on the other hand discovery of biological drugs, enzyme therapy, and bone marrow or solid organ transplantation have improved the hope of treatment and increased life expectancy of patients. Gaucher disease is an IEM and a subgroup of lysosomal storage diseases, which has a wide range presentation. In the last decade, some enzyme replacement therapy for this disease has been developed. Early diagnosis through informing pediatrician and then early ERT can improve life expense, decrease mortality, and morbidity among patients with Gaucher disease. This book tries to be a strike bridge between the sciences of IEMs and clinical practice of pediatrics and adults, through updating all aspects of Gaucher disease and cases presentation by pediatrics and adult practitioners and IEMs experts.

This book represents the contents in six chapters. Chapter 1: Comprehensive review of Gaucher disease pathology, epidemiology, and latest genetic updates. Chapter 2 focuses on clinical manifestations of Gaucher disease. Chapters 3, 4, and 5 are dedicated to diagnosis, initial assessment, current and underdeveloped treatment, and monitoring of treatment. The final chapter is a collection of well-presented patients with Gaucher disease. I hope this book is a useful guide for physicians, especially pediatricians worldwide. I would like to acknowledge the expertise of all contributors and their effort in preparing this book. I also thank ISU ABXIS for their support, and finally, I express my gratitude to the Springer for publishing the book.

Tehran, Iran — Parastoo Rostami

Contents

1 Overview of Lysosomal Storage Diseases (LSDs)

Parastoo Rostami and Maryam Razavi

1.1 Lysosome

1.1.1 Lysosome Structure

Lysosomes were described by the Belgian cytologist Christian René de Duve in the 1950s. Lysosomes are single-membrane-bound organelles found in many human cells. They are small vesicles (ranging in size from 0.1 to 0.5 μm) of fluid, with the lumen's pH about 4.5–5.0 surrounded by a lipid bilaye membrane that helps to keep the enzymes separate from the rest of the cell, protecting the cell from destruction. Typically, a mammalian cell contains around 300 (ranging 50–1000) of this organelle [1] (Fig. 1.1).

Lysosomes have three major components:

- Acid hydrolases and their activators.
- Membrane proteins.
- Lysosomal associated proteins.

Hydrolyzed enzymes of lysosomes are primarily synthesized in the rough endoplasmic reticulum and transported to the Golgi, then they are tagged with the molecule mannose 6-phosphate for import into the lysosome.

P. Rostami (✉) · M. Razavi
Research Center for Growth and Development, Division of Endocrinology and Metabolism, Department of Pediatrics, Pediatrics Center of Excellence, Tehran University of Medical Sciences, Tehran, Iran

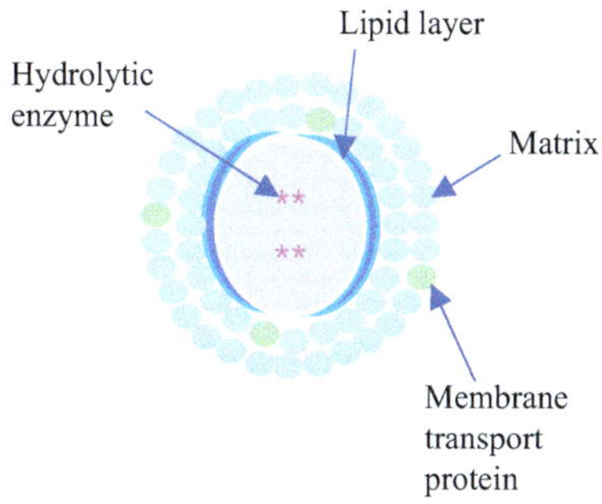

Fig. 1.1 The structure of lysosome

1.1.2 Lysosome Function

Lysosomes are responsible for three vital functions:

- **Digestion of Macromolecules.**
  Lysosomes act as the digestive system which can uptake the degraded material up from inside the cell and hydrolyzed them by more than 60 different hydrolytic enzymes. Enzymes are named for the molecules that they hydrolyze; for example, break down starches into sugars molecule by amylases, proteins into aminoacids by proteases, nucleic acids into nucleotides by nucleases, and lipids into fatty acids and glycerol by lipases. These monomers are recycled and used to synthesize other macromolecules or are released outside the cell as waste products. They also break down and evacuation of unwanted products of the cell [2].

© The Author(s), under exclusive license to Springer Nature Singapore Pte Ltd. 2025

P. Rostami, A. Talea (eds.), *Gaucher Disease*, https://doi.org/10.1007/978-981-96-4763-7_1

- **Intracellular Transport.**
  The lysosome can maintain the cell's internal milieu and digest materials within and outside the cell, in cooperation with the endoplasmic reticulum and Golgi apparatus.
- **Autophagy and Phagocytosis.**
  Lysosomes are involved in autophagy, where they destroy old, damaged, or abnormal proteins and other unwanted substances in the cytoplasm, leading to the recycling of cellular components. Interestingly, lysosomes are involved in other cellular functions, such as apoptosis, plasma membrane repair, secretion, cell signaling, and energy metabolism.
  In phagocytosis, macrophages take up bacteria and viruses (or other pathogens) in phagosomes and fuse them with lysosomes, resulting in the ingestion and destruction of these organisms. In fact, lysosomes have a major role in autoimmunity, antigen presentation, and the regulation of inflammation [3].

1.2 Lysosomal Storage Diseases

1.2.1 Pathophysiology of LSDs

Lysosomal storage diseases (LSDs) are a group of inherited metabolic disorders caused by defects in single genes. Enzyme deficiency is responsible for nearly 70% of these disorders, and the remaining are due to defects in enzyme activators or associated proteins [4].

Lysosome dysfunction leads to the progressive accumulation of degraded substrates and toxic substances within lysosomes. Substrates accumulate in their synthesis sites, such as the spleen, bone, and liver. On the other hand, releasing acid hydrolases into the cytoplasm following lysosome dysfunction leads to cell damage and dysfunction [5, 6]. Apart from genetics, oxidative stress and inflammation processes play important roles in LSDs [7].

1.2.2 Prevalence and Inheritance of LSDs

The exact prevalence of LSDs is difficult to estimate, considering their clinical diversity, which may lead to missed diagnoses. Geography and ethnicity may play important roles in the incidence of LSDs. Although they are individually very rare, their incidence is estimated to be as high as 1 in 4000 in some populations [8].

Most LSDs are inherited in an autosomal recessive pattern, but three disorders have an X-linked inheritance pattern, including Fabry disease, Hunter disease, and Danon disease. In some cases, genotype-phenotype correlations are predictable [7].

1.2.3 Classification of LSDs

Many LSDs have the names of the persons who first described the conditions. Seventy LSDs have been reported so far, and most of these disorders share a common clinical symptom, and all of them are multisystem disorders [9]. LSDs are classified according to the accumulated specific substrate as follows:

- **Mucopolysaccharidoses.**
  - Hurler syndrome.
  - Scheie syndrome.
  - Hurler-Scheie syndrome.
  - Hunter syndrome.
  - Sanfilippo syndrome A, B, C, and D.
  - Morquio syndrome A and B.
  - Maroteaux-Lamy syndrome.
  - Sly syndrome.
- **Sphingolipidoses gangliosidosis.**
  - GM2 gangliosidosis, Sandhoff disease, and Tay-Sachs disease.
  - Niemann-Pick disease A, B, C.
  - Gaucher disease types 1, 2, 3.
  - Metachromatic leukodystrophy.

  - Fabry disease.
  - Krabbe disease.
  - Multiple sulfatase deficiency.
  - GM1 gangliosidosis 1, 2, 3.
  - Oligosaccharidosis.
- **Neuronal ceroid lipofuscinosis (lipofuscin is a waxy pigment).**
  - CLN 1 through CLN 14.
- **Sialic acid disorders (sialic acid).**
- **Mucolipidosis** [10].

1.2.4 Clinical Approach to LSDs

The clinical picture of LSDs varies depending upon the location and extent of storage and can be heterogeneous even within the same disease.

LSDs are heterogeneous in a broad spectrum of clinical manifestations, age of onset, and phenotypic severity [11]. Earlier onset of presentation is associated with more severe symptoms than older age. Some phenotypic clues that raise the suspicion of an LSD include skin changes, coarse facial features, hepatosplenomegaly, skeletal abnormalities, scoliosis, finger contractures, gaze palsy, ataxia, etc. [6].

1.2.5 Laboratory Approach to LSDs

Given the clinical heterogeneity in LSDs, clinical suspicion must be followed by routine-specific biochemical tests. The first step in the diagnostic approach to LSDs consists of qualitative and quantitative urinary analyses for specific undegraded macromolecules (Fig. 1.2):

- Quantitative analysis of glycosaminoglycans (GAGs) by a dye-binding assay, followed by electrophoresis, can detect and differentiate the type of GAGs.
- A urine oligosaccharide assay can detect urine sugars using the thin-layer or high-pressure liquid chromatography method.
- Urine-free sialic acid concentration can be measured through mass spectrometry [10].

Although assessing urine metabolites is recommended as a first-line diagnosis for LSDs, this test can only detect some patients, and individual carriers may be missed due to false-negative results. Therefore, if strongly suspected, normal urinary screens should still be followed by enzyme analysis [12].

Other biochemical tests, such as serum creatine kinase (CK) or chitotriosidase, can be elevated in Pompe disease or Gaucher (may be Niemann-Pick C disease), respectively. All positive results still need to be confirmed by specific enzyme assays and/or molecular analyses. Skin fibroblasts are the preferred cells for enzyme activity measurement because of maximal in these cells enzyme activity but leucocytes have other isoenzymes that may interfere to assay [12, 13].

1.2.6 Other Techniques for the Specific Diagnosis of LSDs

Some LSDs need additional tests for more investigation, such as the following:

- Abdominal sonography.
- Brain MRI.
- X-rays.
- Pulmonary function tests.
- Echocardiogram (EKG).
- Renal and liver function.
- Audiometry assessment.
- Visual examination.
- Hemogram [14].

1.2.7 Newborn Screening Techniques

Lysosomal storage disorders should be included in the newborn screening program (NBS) because effective treatments are available for some of these diseases, so early diagnosis and treatment will improve the outcomes of patients. Several methods have been proposed for NBS, including

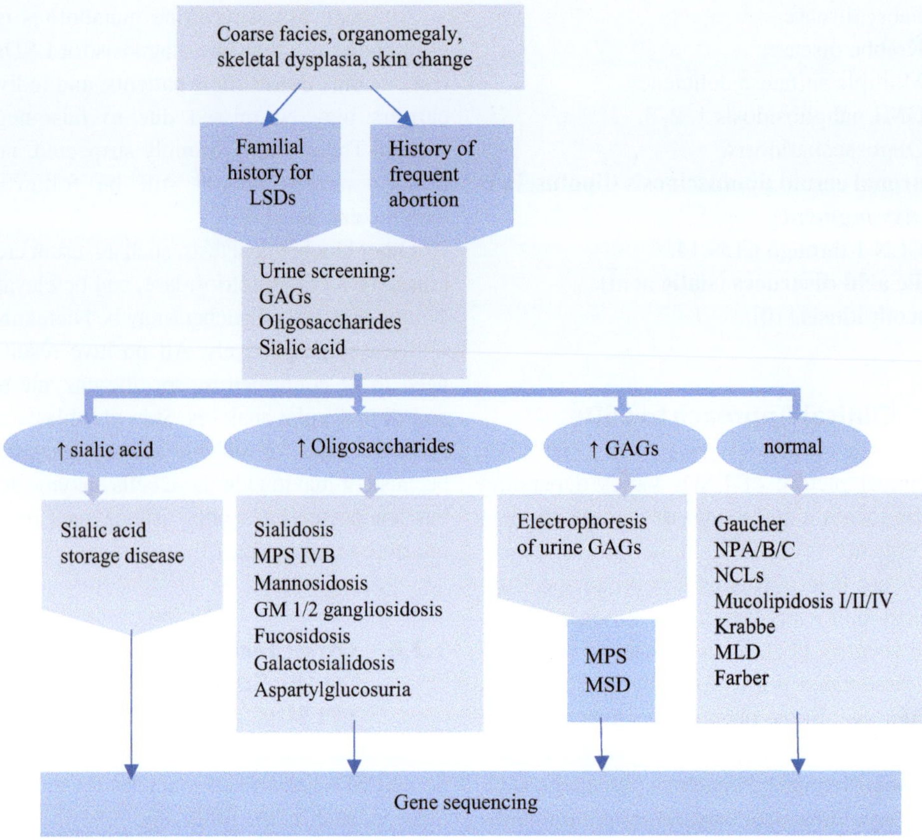

Fig. 1.2 Biochemical diagnostic algorithm of LSDs. *GAGs* glycosaminoglycans, *MLD* metachromatic leukodystrophy, *MPS* mucopolysaccharidosis, *MSD* multiple sulfatase deficiency, *NPA/B* Niemann Pick type A/B, *NPC* Niemann Pick type C, *NCL* neuronal ceroid lipofuscinosis

direct enzymatic activity assays (using the tandem mass spectrometry method or fluorometric method), lysosomal biomarker assays, lysosomal protein abundance assays, and lysosomal enzyme gene sequencing. A positive NBS result should be confirmed by a molecular study because of the probability of false positive results [14, 15].

1.2.8 Carrier Screening

The detection of carriers of LSDs in certain populations with a high risk of these disorders allows couples to be informed about the risk of LSDs in their offspring to guide decision-making on marriage and reproduction in these populations, as well as allow for prenatal testing [16].

1.2.9 Prenatal Screening

Prenatal screening through chorionic villus biopsy and/or amniocentesis is available for many inborn errors of metabolism, including LSDs. This approach allows physicians and families to detect affected fetuses and plan for treatment [12].

1.2.10 Treatment of LSDs

The treatment/management of LSDs should be under the supervision of multiple disciplines. Improvements in treatment for these patients have increased their life expectancy [17]. Treatment options based on specific substrate accumulation includes the following:

- Enzyme replacement therapy.
- Chaperone therapy.
- Substrate reduction therapy.
- Small-molecule-assisted substrate transportation.
- Proteostasis Regulators.
- Anti-inflammatory Agent.
- Hematopoietic stem cell transplantation.
- Gene therapy [14].

Learning Point

- Lysosomes have a critical role in the degradation of substrates.
- Lysosome dysfunction causes the accumulation of degraded materials in the cell, leading to organ enlargement and cellular dysfunction.
- Lysosomal storage diseases (LSDs) present with a variety of phenotypes.
- Diagnosis of LSDs is confirmed by enzyme assays and molecular tests.
- Early diagnosis and management of LSDs through NBS is necessary.
- There are several treatments available for LSDs.

References

1. Sabatini DD, Adesnik MB. The biogenesis of membranes and organelles. In: Beaudet AL, Vogelstein B, Kinzler KW, Antonarakis SE, Ballabio A, Gibson KM, Mitchell G, editors. The online metabolic and molecular bases of inherited disease. New York: McGraw-Hill; 2014.
2. Lawrence RE, Zoncu R. The lysosome as a cellular centre for signalling, metabolism and quality control. Nat Cell Biol. 2019;21:133–42.
3. Finkbeiner S. The autophagy lysosomal pathway and neurodegeneration. Cold Spring Harb Perspect Biol. 2020; 12(3).
4. Valle D, Beaudet AL, Vogelstein B, Kinzler KW, Antonarakis SE, Ballabio A, Gibson K, Mitchell G. The online metabolic and molecular bases of inherited disease. New York: McGraw-Hill; 2014.
5. Stirnemann J, Belmatoug N, Camou F, Serratrice C, Froissart R, Caillaud C, Levade T, Astudillo L, Serratrice J, Brassier A, Rose C, Billette de Villemeur T, Berger MG. A review of Gaucher disease pathophysiology, clinical presentation and treatments. Int J Mol Sci. 2017;17(2):18.
6. Ballabio A, Bonifacino JS. Lysosomes as dynamic regulators of cell and organismal homeostasis. Nat Rev Mol Cell Biol. 2020;21(2):101–18.
7. Donida B, Jacques CED, Mescka CP, Rodrigues DGB, Marchetti DP, Ribas G, Giugliani R, Vargas CR. Oxidative damage and redox in lysosomal storage disorders: biochemical markers. Clin Chim Acta. 2017;466:46–53.
8. Giugliani R, Vairo F, Beck M, Wraith E, Cowan T, Grabowski G. Lysosomal disorders. In: Sarafoglou K, Hoffmann GF, Roth KS, editors. Pediatric endocrinology and inborn errors of metabolism. 2nd ed. New York: McGraw-Hill Education; 2017b. p. 983–1021.
9. Platt FM, d'Azzo A, Davidson BL, Neufeld EF, Tifft CJ. Lysosomal storage diseases. Nat Rev Dis Primers. 2018;4(1):27.
10. Leal AF, Nieto WG, Candelo E, Pachajoa H, Alméciga-Díaz CJ. Hematological findings in lysosomal storage disorders: a perspective from the medical laboratory. J Int Fed Clin Chem. 2022;33:28–42.
11. Kingma SDK, Bodamer OA, Wijburg FA. Epidemiology and diagnosis of lysosomal storage disorders; challenges of screening. Best Pract Res Clin Endocrinol Metab. 2015;29(2):145–57.
12. Filocamo M, Morrone A. Lysosomal storage disorders: molecular basis and laboratory testing. Hum Genomics. 2011;5(3):156–69.
13. Mokhtariye A, Hagh-Nazari L, Varasteh AR, Keyfi F. Diagnostic methods for lysosomal storage disease. Rep Biochem Mol Biol. 2019;7(2):119–28.
14. Rajkumar V, Dumpa V. Lysosomal storage disease. StatPearls: online [internet]. Last update, July 24, 2023.
15. Elliott S, Buroker N, Cournoyer JJ, Potier AM, Trometer JD, et al. Pilot study of newborn screening for six lysosomal storage diseases using tandem mass spectrometry. Mol Genet Metab. 2016;118(4):304–9.
16. Kaback M, Lim-Steele J, Zeiger K. Tay-Sachs disease- carrier screening, prenatal diagnosis, and the molecular era: an international perspective, 1970 to 1993. J AM Med Accos. 1993;270(19):2307–15.
17. Wenger DA, Coppola S, Liu S-L. Insights into the diagnosis and treatment of lysosomal storage diseases. Arch Neurol. 2003;60(3):322–8.

Overview of Gaucher Disease 2

Saeedeh Saeedi, Reihaneh Mohsenipour, and Parastoo Rostami

2.1 Introduction

Sphingolipids are found in all mammalian cell membranes and in plasma lipoproteins. They act as structural and functional (numerous biological/physiological functions) elements. The cornerstone of sphingolipids is long-chain sphingosine, which can be N-acylated by different fatty acids (mainly palmitoyl-CoA), leading to ceramide formation (Fig. 2.1).

Ceramide can be synthesized through two pathways: [1] the de novo pathway (in the endoplasmic reticulum), from palmitate and serine (Fig. 2.2a), and [2] the salvage pathway (Fig. 2.2b) [1].

Sphingolipids are categorized into two main classes based on their head group:

- Phosphosphingolipids (PSLs).
- Glycosphingolipids (GSLs).

PSLs include the addition of one or more phosphate groups to the sphingolipid. Sphingomyelin is the most common PSL, consisting of phosphocholine or phosphoethanolamine and ceramide, which is a major component of myelin (Fig. 2.3a).

Glycosphingolipids are made of a ceramide bound to at least one carbohydrate (Fig. 2.3b). Neutral GSLs mainly serve as simple biosynthetic precursors for more complex derivatives, and they are classified into three major groups:

- Galactosylceramide (also called galactocerebroside) (GalCer).
- Glucosylceramide (also called glucocerebroside) (GlcCer).
- Lactosylceramide (LacCer) [2]

Glycosphingolipids and phosphosphingolipids are removed from the plasma membrane and transported to the lysosomes for degradation via the endolysosomal pathway.

Complex glycosphingolipids are degraded to

- Galactosylceramide and.
- Glucosylceramide (Fig. 2.4).

These lipids are then catalyzed by beta-glucosidase and beta-galactosidase to regenerate ceramide. Sphingomyelin is hydrolyzed by sphingomyelinase to form ceramide [3].

Sphingolipidoses are inherited metabolic disorders caused by defects in the lysosomal enzymes involved in sphingolipid degradation, leading to the accumulation of nondegradable

S. Saeedi
Clinical Biochemistry, Metabolic Disorders Research Center, Endocrinology and Metabolism Molecular-Cellular Sciences Institute, Tehran University of Medical Sciences, Tehran, Iran

R. Mohsenipour · P. Rostami (✉)
Research Center for Growth and Development, Division of Endocrinology and Metabolism, Department of Pediatrics, Pediatrics Center of Excellence, Tehran University of Medical Sciences, Tehran, Iran

© The Author(s), under exclusive license to Springer Nature Singapore Pte Ltd. 2025
P. Rostami, A. Talea (eds.), *Gaucher Disease*, https://doi.org/10.1007/978-981-96-4763-7_2

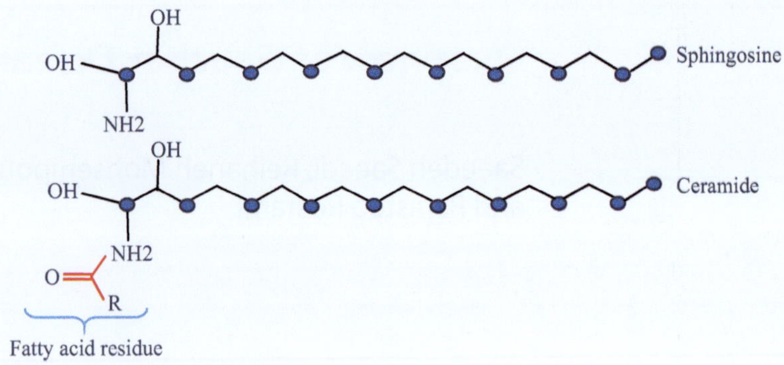

Fig. 2.1 Structure of sphingosine and ceramide

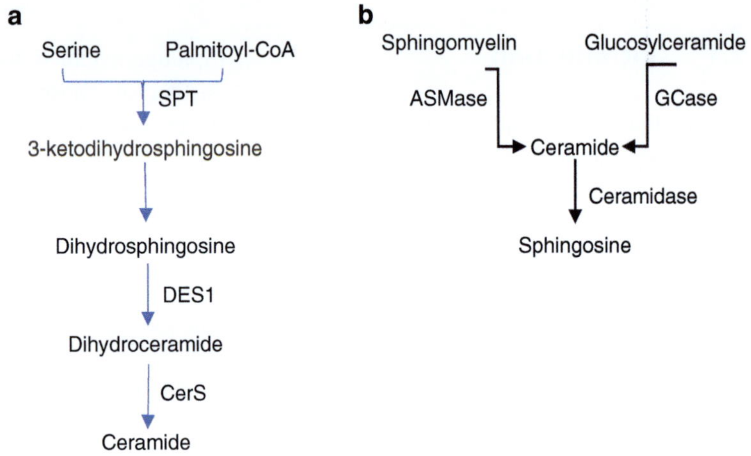

Fig. 2.2 (**a**) De novo sphingolipid synthesis pathways. *SPT* serine palmitoyl-CoA transferase, *CerS* ceramide synthase, *DES1* desaturase. (**b**) Salvage sphingolipid synthesis pathway. *GCase* glucosylceramidase, *ASMase* acid sphingomyelinase

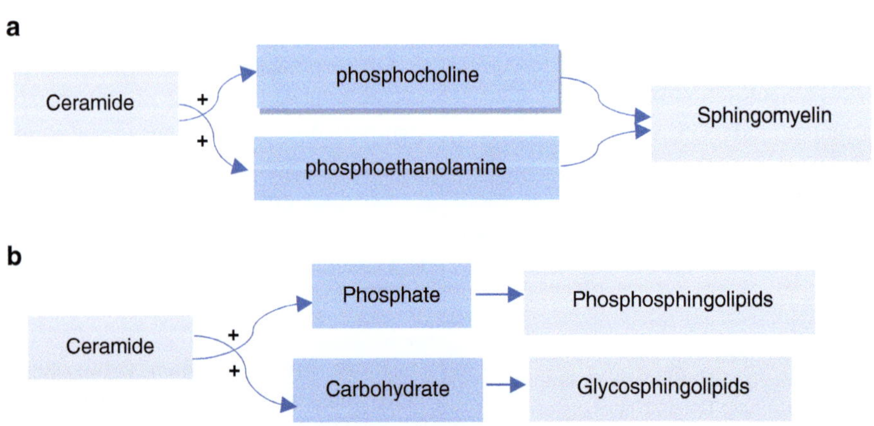

Fig. 2.3 (**a**) The pathway of sphingomyelin synthesis and (**b**) phosphosphingolipid and glycosphingolipid synthesis

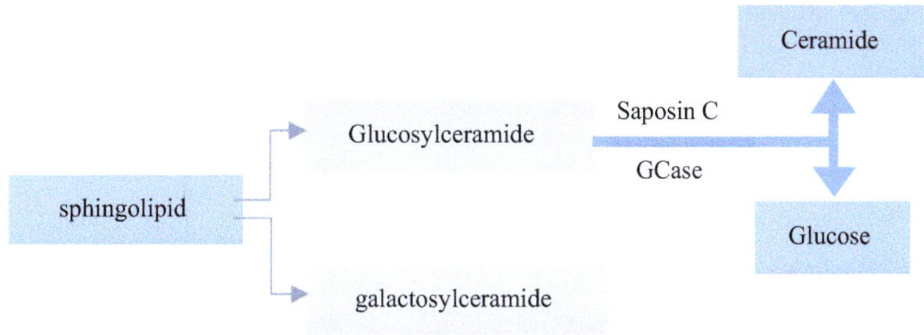

Fig. 2.4 Hydrolysis pathway of glucosylceramide (GlcCer) by glucocerebrosidase (GCase) in the lysosome

substrates in the organs. Disorders of sphingolipid synthesis are caused by mutations in the genes encoding the enzymes, activators, and transporters [4].

2.2 Epidemiology

Gaucher disease (GD) was first explained by Philippe Gaucher in 1882 in a patient with massive splenomegaly without leukemia [5]. It is the most frequent lysosomal storage disease. Type 1 GD (GD1) is the most common in Europe, Israel, and the United States.

Interestingly, type 1 GD is common in the Ashkenazi Jewish population, but type 2 GD (GD2) affects all ethnicities. A recent report estimated the incidence of GD in the general population to be between 0.4 and 5.8 per 100,000, with a prevalence of 0.7 to 1.8 per 100,000 [6]. The carrier frequency in the Ashkenazi Jewish population is approximately 1 in 12 [7].

The estimated incidence of GD2 (or acute neuronopathic GD) is about 1 in 150,000 [8]. The incidence of type 3 GD (or subacute or chronic neuronopathic GD) is 1 in 200,000, but its prevalence is considerably greater than that of GD2 due to the increased survival rate of GD3 patients. GD3 occurs in all ethnic groups but may be more prevalent in East Asia, northern Europe, and Egypt [9].

2.3 Pathophysiology

Gaucher disease (GD) (OMIM#230800) is an autosomal recessive inborn error of metabolism caused by a deficiency of the enzyme acid β-glucosidase (glucocerebrosidase or glucosylceramidase), which leads to increased 20-100-fold increase in the level of glucosylceramide in the liver, spleen, kidneys, lungs, brain, and bone marrow. Some mechanisms that have been suggested in the pathogenesis of GD include (Fig. 2.5) the following.

2.3.1 Degraded Substrate Accumulation

- Glucosylceramide can be stored in the macrophages, inducing their transformation into Gaucher cells [5, 10]. Under a light microscope, Gaucher cells are enlarged, with eccentric nuclei, condensed chromatin, and cytoplasm that has a heterogeneous "crumpled tissue paper" appearance (Fig. 2.6). These characteristics are related to the accumulation of GlcCer in cells [5]. The signs and symptoms of GD are due to the accumulation of lipid-rich macrophages in the reticuloendothelial system, including the liver, spleen, bone marrow, bone, and other organs. The accumulation of lipid-rich macrophages accounts for less than 2% of the mass in the liver, spleen, and other organs. Therefore, it is assumed that additional factors, such as inflammatory response and hyperplastic cellularity, may be attributed to organ weight and volume [11].

2.3.2 Dysfunction of Other Proteins

- The protein saposin C presents glucocerebroside to glucocerebroside and activates the enzyme. In addition, lysosomal integral mem-

Fig. 2.5 Medullary smear showing Gaucher cells with plasma cells with a "crumpled tissue paper" appearance in a patient with Gaucher disease [5]

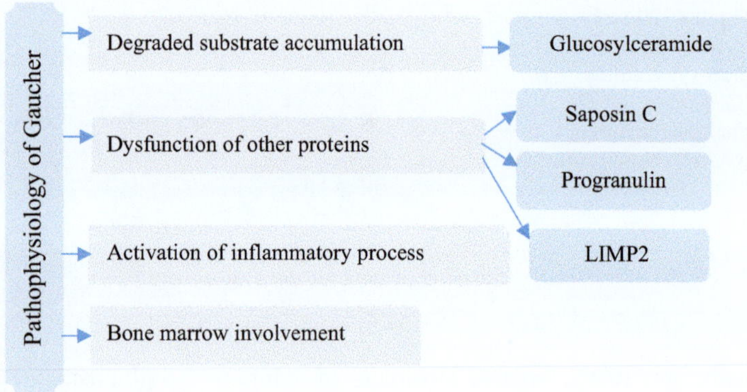

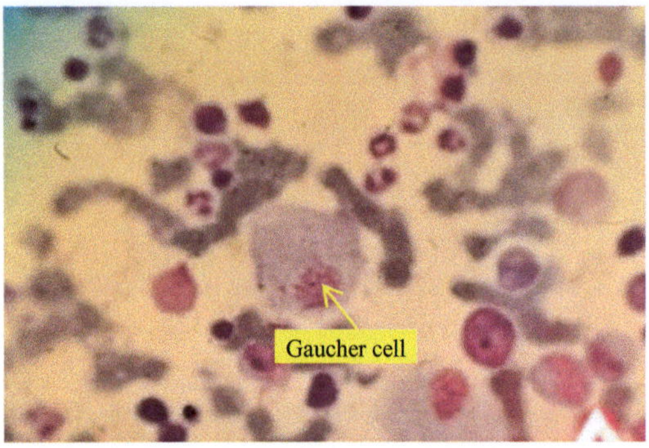

Fig. 2.6 Different mechanisms in the pathophysiology of Gaucher disease

brane protein (LIMP2) is involved in transporting glucocerebroside to the lysosome, so maybe there is a relationship between the dysfunctions of these proteins and GD [12, 13].
- Progranulin (PGRN) can act as a cochaperone for the lysosomal localization of glucocerebrosidase in pathological states, linking glucocerebrosidase to heat shock protein 70 (HSP70). The insufficiency of this protein is associated with GD, and it could be used as a new treatment in the future [14–16].

2.3.3 Activation of the Inflammatory Process

- Gaucher cells and macrophages induce the overexpression and secretion of lysosomal proteases such as cathepsins, inflammatory chemokines such as interleukin (IL6, IL-8, and IL-10), macrophage inflammatory proteins (MIP: 1-alpha and 1-beta), and chemotactic factors cysteine-X-cysteine motif chemokine ligand (CXCL 2, 9, 10, and 11) [11, 17–22]. The activation of complement C5a and C5a receptor 1 (C5aR1) may be involved in chemotaxis and Gaucher cell aggregation [23].
- "Alternatively activated" macrophage is a secretory phenotype of Gaucher cells, which is often associated with chronic inflammation, healing, and fibrosis [24].
- The level of deacylated glucosylceramide, glucosylsphingosine, is increased in the brain in patients with neuronopathic types of GD, and it is supposed to have a role in the pathogenesis of neurologic involvement. This substrate may stimulate inflammation, gammopathy, and neurotoxicity [25].

2.3.4 Bone Marrow Involvement

- Bone involvement in GD1 includes decreased mineral density, marrow infiltration, and infarction. The exact mechanisms of decreased bone mineral density are unknown. Patients with GD cannot achieve peak bone mass and have impaired osteoclast regulation or overproduction of cytokines by activated macrophages. The presence of fibrosis and osteosclerosis in the bone marrow leads to a decrease in the capacity of hematopoiesis [26].

2.4 Genetics

2.4.1 *GBA1* Gene Characteristics

GD is an autosomal recessive genetic disease caused by mutations in the glucosylceramidase beta 1 (*GBA1*) gene, mapped on chromosome 1 (1q21), and is approximately 7.5 kb long and contains 11 exons. A highly homologous 5.5 kb pseudogene has been located 16 kb downstream from the active gene (Fig. 2.7).

A pathogenic variant in the *GBA1* gene leads to significantly decreased activity of the glucocerebrosidase, which hydrolyzes glucosylceramide (GlcCer) into ceramide and glucose [5].

At least 495 variants are listed in the Human Gene Mutation Database for the *GBA1* gene, with about 80% of these variants being single-nucleotide substitutions [27]. Other pathogenic variants include deletions, insertions, and other complex alleles [28]. Germline mutations and uniparental disomy are also described in GD [29, 30].

Three frequent variants have been reported:

- The missense variant c.1226A > G allele (N370S or p.N409S) has some residual enzyme activity [31]. There is a genotype-phenotype correlation in which the presence of the c.1226A > G variant in a homozygous or compound heterozygous form leads to GD1 rather than a neurologic phenotype [7]. The c.1226A > G variant is common in non-Jewish Europeans and Ashkenazi Jews but is rare in Asian populations [32].
- The variant c.1448 T > C allele (L444P or p. L483P) is the most common mutant allele worldwide, which accounts for 18% of the alleles. It has been described in northern Sweden and Northern Europe. A homozygous c.1448 T > C allele is related to a severe phenotype, often with GD3, but the phenotype can be highly variable. On the other hand, a heterozygous c.1448 T > C allele is associated with GD2 [33]. The variant L444P appears to be the most common in India, which occurs in the pseudogene sequence and is associated with extreme variation ranging from lethal collodion skin baby phenotype to GD3 phenotype with minimal oculomotor apraxia [35]. The most prevalent genotype in Egyptian patients with GD3 is homozygous p. Leu483Pro, followed by homozygous p. Asp448His [34].
- The second most common pathogenic variant in Ashkenazi Jews with GD is the c.84dupG allele (c.84insG mutation), which accounts for about 7% of mutant alleles. It is a null variant, and affected patients are compound heterozygotes and related to any of the three types of GD. Homozygotes have not been reported because of prenatal lethality [31].

Although GD is an autosomal recessive disorder, there are exceptions to the conventional Mendelian pattern of inheritance, such as new mutations or uniparental disomy [37]. Some

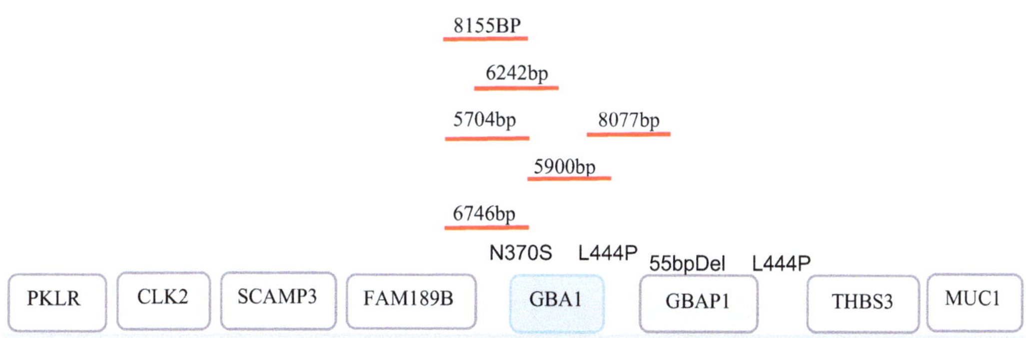

Fig. 2.7 *GBA1* gene, mapped on chromosome 1 (1q21) with approximately 7.5 kb in length and containing 11 exons

patients with GD2 and unrelated parents with de novo or germline mutations on the maternal allele have been reported [38].

A patient with GD3 and uniparental disomy of chromosome 1 was reported in a proband with a concurrent Charcot-Marie-Tooth disease, who was homozygous for both L444P (p.L483P) in *GBA1* and S78L in *MPZ* (myelin protein zero) [29].

In Mendelian disorders, somatic mosaicism may occur. This was described in a patient with GD2 who had been found to have genotype L444P/N370S at first, but further investigation revealed that the actual genotype was L444P/N370S + S488P, where S488P (p.S527P) was found to be a somatic mutation [39].

There are two mutations on the same allele in some situations of GD. One patient with the genotype N370S/ N370S also carried the mutation L444P [40], and another patient with GD2 and the genotype G202R/G202R (p.G241Rp./G241R) carried M361I (M400I) as well [41].

Learning Points

- Gaucher disease is a lysosomal storage disorder.
- Pathogenic variants in the *GBA1* gene cause all forms of Gaucher disease.
- The accumulation of glucosylceramide results in cellular dysfunction and visceromegaly, while dysfunction of other proteins (saposin C, progranulin, lysosomal integral membrane protein-2 (LIMP2)) and inflammatory processes also play a role in the disease's pathophysiology.
- A genotype-phenotype correlation has been confirmed for certain variants.
- Three frequent variants in the *GBA1* gene include the missense variant c.1226A > G allele (N370S or p.N409S), the variant c.1448 T > C allele (L444P or p.L483P), and the c.84dupG allele (c.84insG mutation).

2.5 Summary

The c.1226A > G, c.84dupG, IVS2 + 1G > A, and c.1448 T > C pathogenic variants account for 93% of alleles in Ashkenazi patients [32].

The c.1226A > G and c.1448 T > C variants together account for approximately 70% of mutant alleles in non-Ashkenazi European patients [33]. The c.1448T variant is encountered worldwide. Mutant allele frequencies are different in Asian populations [35].

The variant L444P appears to be the most common in India, occurring in the pseudogene sequence and associated with an extreme variation range, from lethal collodion skin baby phenotype to GD3 phenotype with minimal oculomotor apraxia [36]. The most prevalent genotype in Egyptian patients with GD3 is homozygous p.Leu483Pro, followed by homozygous p.Asp448His [34].

References

1. Astudillo L, Sabourdy F, Therville N, Bode H, Ségui B, Andrieu-Abadie N, et al. Human genetic disorders of sphingolipid biosynthesis. J Inherit Metab Dis. 2015;38(1):65–76.
2. Pasquet L, Camara K, Bloom AC, Richardson SK, Howell AR, Terabe M, et al. The ceramide structure of sulfatide-analogues influences the functional activity of type II NKT cells. J Immunol. 2018;200(1 Supplement):57.20.
3. Mullen TD, Hannun YA, Obeid LM. Ceramide synthases at the centre of sphingolipid metabolism and biology. Biochem J. 2012;441(3):789–802.
4. Kolter T, Sandhoff K. Sphingolipid metabolism diseases. Biochim Biophys Acta. 2006;1758(12):2057–79.
5. Stirnemann J, Belmatoug N, Camou F, Serratrice C, Froissart R, Caillaud C, et al. A review of Gaucher disease pathophysiology, clinical presentation and treatments. Int J Mol Sci. 2017;18(2)
6. Nalysnyk L, Rotella P, Simeone JC, Hamed A, Weinreb N. Gaucher disease epidemiology and natural

history: a comprehensive review of the literature. Hematology. 2017;22(2):65–73.
7. Koprivica V, Stone DL, Park JK, Callahan M, Frisch A, Cohen IJ, et al. Analysis and classification of 304 mutant alleles in patients with type 1 and type 3 Gaucher disease. Am J Hum Genet. 2000;66(6):1777–86.
8. Sidransky E. New perspectives in type 2 Gaucher disease. Adv Pediatr Infect Dis. 1997;44:73–107.
9. ylki-Szymańska A, Vellodi A, El-Beshlawy A, Cole JA, Kolodny E. Neuronopathic Gaucher disease: demographic and clinical features of 131 patients enrolled in the international collaborative Gaucher group neurological outcomes subregistry. J Inherit Metab Dis. 2010;33(4):339–46.
10. Svennerholm L, Håkansson G, Månsson JE, Nilsson O. Chemical differentiation of the Gaucher subtypes. Prog Clin Biol Res. 1982;95:231–52.
11. Cox TM. Gaucher disease: understanding the molecular pathogenesis of sphingolipidoses. J Inherit Metab Dis. 2001;24(Suppl 2):106–21. discussion 87-8
12. Grabowski GA, Antommaria AHM, Kolodny EH, Mistry PK. Gaucher disease: basic and translational science needs for more complete therapy and management. Mol Genet Metab. 2021;132(2):59–75.
13. Tamargo RJ, Velayati A, Goldin E, Sidransky E. The role of saposin C in Gaucher disease. Mol Genet Metab. 2012;106(3):257–63.
14. Jian J, Tian QY, Hettinghouse A, Zhao S, Liu H, Wei J, et al. Progranulin recruits HSP70 to β-Glucocerebrosidase and is therapeutic against Gaucher disease. EBioMedicine. 2016;13:212–24.
15. Jian J, Zhao S, Tian QY, Liu H, Zhao Y, Chen WC, et al. Association between Progranulin and Gaucher disease. EBioMedicine. 2016;11:127–37.
16. Tayebi N, Lopez G, Do J, Sidransky E, Pro-cathepsin D. Prosaposin, and Progranulin: lysosomal networks in parkinsonism. Trends Mol Med. 2020;26(10):913–23.
17. Allen MJ, Myer BJ, Khokher AM, Rushton N, Cox TM. Pro-inflammatory cytokines and the pathogenesis of Gaucher's disease: increased release of interleukin-6 and interleukin-10. QJM. 1997;90(1):19–25.
18. Hollak CE, Evers L, Aerts JM, van Oers MH. Elevated levels of M-CSF, sCD14 and IL8 in type 1 Gaucher disease. Blood Cells Mol Dis. 1997;23(2):201–12.
19. Mistry PK, Liu J, Yang M, Nottoli T, McGrath J, Jain D, et al. Glucocerebrosidase gene-deficient mouse recapitulates Gaucher disease displaying cellular and molecular dysregulation beyond the macrophage. Proc Natl Acad Sci USA. 2010;107(45):19473–8.
20. Moran MT, Schofield JP, Hayman AR, Shi GP, Young E, Cox TM. Pathologic gene expression in Gaucher disease: up-regulation of cysteine proteinases including osteoclastic cathepsin K. Blood. 2000;96(5):1969–78.
21. Pandey MK, Jabre NA, Xu YH, Zhang W, Setchell KD, Grabowski GA. Gaucher disease: chemotactic factors and immunological cell invasion in a mouse model. Mol Genet Metab. 2014;111(2):163–71.
22. Pavlova EV, Deegan PB, Tindall J, McFarlane I, Mehta A, Hughes D, et al. Potential biomarkers of osteonecrosis in Gaucher disease. Blood Cells Mol Dis. 2011;46(1):27–33.
23. Pandey MK, Burrow TA, Rani R, Martin LJ, Witte D, Setchell KD, et al. Complement drives glucosylceramide accumulation and tissue inflammation in Gaucher disease. Nature. 2017;543(7643):108–12.
24. Gordon S. Macrophage heterogeneity and tissue lipids. J Clin Invest. 2007;117(1):89–93.
25. Schueler UH, Kolter T, Kaneski CR, Blusztajn JK, Herkenham M, Sandhoff K, et al. Toxicity of glucosylsphingosine (glucopsychosine) to cultured neuronal cells: a model system for assessing neuronal damage in Gaucher disease type 2 and 3. Neurobiol Dis. 2003;14(3):595–601.
26. Reed M, Baker RJ, Mehta AB, Hughes DA. Enhanced differentiation of osteoclasts from mononuclear precursors in patients with Gaucher disease. Blood Cells Mol Dis. 2013;51(3):185–94.
27. Hruska KS, LaMarca ME, Scott CR, Sidransky E. Gaucher disease: mutation and polymorphism spectrum in the glucocerebrosidase gene (GBA). Hum Mutat. 2008;29(5):567–83.
28. Montfort M, Chabás A, Vilageliu L, Grinberg D. Functional analysis of 13 GBA mutant alleles identified in Gaucher disease patients: pathogenic changes and "modifier" polymorphisms. Hum Mutat. 2004;23(6):567–75.
29. Benko WS, Hruska KS, Nagan N, Goker-Alpan O, Hart PS, Schiffmann R, et al. Uniparental disomy of chromosome 1 causing concurrent Charcot-Marie-Tooth and Gaucher disease type 3. Neurology. 2008;70(12):976–8.
30. Zampieri S, Cattarossi S, Bembi B, Dardis A. GBA analysis in next-generation era: pitfalls, challenges, and possible solutions. J Mol Diagn. 2017;19(5):733–41.
31. Charrow J, Andersson HC, Kaplan P, Kolodny EH, Mistry P, Pastores G, et al. The Gaucher registry: demographics and disease characteristics of 1698 patients with Gaucher disease. Arch Intern Med. 2000;160(18):2835–43.
32. Beutler E, Nguyen NJ, Henneberger MW, Smolec JM, McPherson RA, West C, et al. Gaucher disease: gene frequencies in the Ashkenazi Jewish population. Am J Hum Genet. 1993;52(1):85–8.
33. Alfonso P, Cenarro A, Pérez-Calvo JI, Giralt M, Giraldo P, Pocoví M. Mutation prevalence among 51 unrelated Spanish patients with Gaucher disease: identification of 11 novel mutations. Blood Cells Mol Dis. 2001;27(5):882–91.
34. El-Beshlawy A, Abdel-Azim K, Abdel-Salam A, Selim YMM, Said F, Gebril NA, et al. Egyptian Gaucher disease type 3 patients: a large cohort study spanning two decades. J Rare Dis. 2023;2(1):7.
35. Jeong SY, Park SJ, Kim HJ. Clinical and genetic characteristics of Korean patients with Gaucher disease. Blood Cells Mol Dis. 2011;46(1):11–4.

36. Ankleshwaria C, Mistri M, Bavdekar A, Muranjan M, Dave U, Tamhankar P, et al. Novel mutations in the glucocerebrosidase gene of Indian patients with Gaucher disease. J Hum Genet. 2014;59(4):223–8.
37. Nakka P, Pattillo Smith S, O'Donnell-Luria AH, McManus KF, Mountain JL, Ramachandran S, et al. Characterization of prevalence and health consequences of uniparental Disomy in four million individuals from the general population. Am J Hum Genet. 2019;105(5):921–32.
38. Saranjam H, Chopra SS, Levy H, Stubblefield BK, Maniwang E, Cohen IJ, et al. A germline or de novo mutation in two families with Gaucher disease: implications for recessive disorders. Eur J Hum Genet. 2013;21(1):115–7.
39. Filocamo M, Bonuccelli G, Mazzotti R, Corsolini F, Stroppiano M, Regis S, et al. Somatic mosaicism in a patient with Gaucher disease type 2: implication for genetic counseling and therapeutic decision-making. Blood Cells Mol Dis. 2000;26(6):611–2.
40. Beutler E, Liebman H, Gelbart T, Stefanski E. Three Gaucher-disease-producing mutations in a patient with Gaucher disease: mechanism and diagnostic implications. Acta Haematol. 2000;104(2–3):103–5.
41. Siebert M, Bock H, Michelin-Tirelli K, Coelho JC, Giugliani R, Saraiva-Pereira ML. Novel mutations in the glucocerebrosidase gene of brazilian patients with Gaucher disease. JIMD Rep. 2013;9:7–16.

3 Overview of Clinical Presentation: Pathologic and Radiologic Findings of Gaucher Disease

Reza Shervin Badv, Zahra Rezaei, and Parastoo Rostami

3.1 Introduction

Gaucher disease (GD), like other lysosomal storage disorders, is a multisystem disease. Beta glucosidase deficiency leads to the progressive intralysosomal accumulation of glucosylceramide and other degraded substrates, causing cell damage and dysfunction. The exact cause of GD remains unknown despite the identification of the exact pathologic and genetic causes of the disease. Clinical heterogenicity results in variability of signs and symptoms among patients with the same mutation. On the contrary, patients with the same clinical manifestations may have very different genetic mutations. Therefore, a broad spectrum of presentation severity, from perinatal lethal to asymptomatic disease, is expected [1].

R. S. Badv
Pediatric Neurology Division, Ataxia Clinic, Pediatrics Center of Excellence, Tehran University of Medical Sciences, Tehran, Iran

Z. Rezaei
Pediatric and Adolescence Multidisciplinary Research Center (PAMERC), Pediatrics Center of Excellence, Tehran University of Medical Sciences, Tehran, Iran

P. Rostami (✉)
Research Center for Growth and Development, Division of Endocrinology and Metabolism, Department of Pediatrics, Pediatrics Center of Excellence, Tehran University of Medical Sciences, Tehran, Iran

3.2 Clinical Classification of GD

GD may present at any age, from fetal to childhood or adulthood. It is classified into three major forms according to the presence or absence of neurological manifestation: GD type 1 (GD1), GD type 2 (GD2), and GD type 3(GD3). Perinatal and lethal forms and cardiovascular diseases are included in GD1 and GD3, respectively. There is an overlap among and within the forms of GD, indicating that GD is a continuum of manifestations rather than three distinct subtypes [1, 2]. GD1 is differentiated from GD2 (acute neuropathic) and GD3 (chronic neuropathic) by the lack of neurologic involvement (Fig. 3.1) [3].

Gaucher Disease Type1 (GD1)
GD1 is defined by the lack of neurological symptoms and accounts for about 90% of all cases in the Western world. It can be present at any age (median age: 10–20 years old) [3], and there is a variation in the clinical presentation, severity, and course of the disease, even among other affected siblings [4]. A study reported anemia and hepatosplenomegaly as the most common clinical manifestations of 887 patients with GD1 diagnosed by age 6 years, but bone involvement was more prevalent in patients who were diagnosed through teenage years [5]. Additionally, many childhood patients experienced growth retardation, bone crises, and thrombocytopenia [6]. The signs and symptoms of GD1 include the following.

© The Author(s), under exclusive license to Springer Nature Singapore Pte Ltd. 2025
P. Rostami, A. Talea (eds.), *Gaucher Disease*, https://doi.org/10.1007/978-981-96-4763-7_3

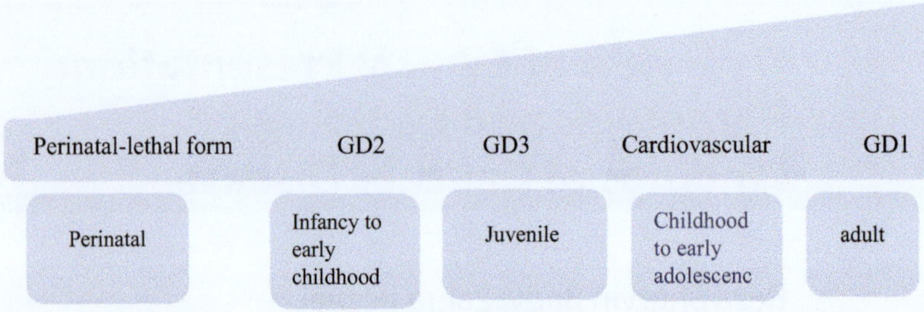

Fig. 3.1 Spectrum clinical phenotypes of Gaucher disease according to age and the severity of the disease

General Signs and Symptoms

- Fatigue is common (half of patients) and can affect daily activities.
- In children, growth retardation and delayed puberty commonly occur, resulting in the stature and weight being less than fifth percentile in 34% of patients [5].

Visceromegaly

- Splenomegaly is the most common presenting sign and occurs in more than 90% of patients.
- The spleen enlarges to an average of 15.2 times its normal size [3].
- The liver size increases in 60–80% of patients but less than the spleen.
- Splenic infarction and spontaneous rupture occur very rarely, which leads to acute abdominal pain and unnecessary surgery [7].
- Liver size increases to as much as two to three times its normal size for age [3].
- Hepatic cirrhosis and fibrosis are rare.
- Hepatic failure and portal hypertension are uncommon [8].
- Gaucheroma may be presented as a focal lesion in the liver and spleen and occurs in 40% of GD1 patients.
- This lesion must be differentiated from hepatocellular carcinoma or lymphoma of the spleen [9].
- Gallstones, especially cholesterol and GlcCer stones, are five times higher than in the general population [10].

Bleeding Tendency

Bleeding propensity in patients with GD1 is related to

- Usually, thrombocytopenia (60–90% of cases).
- Sometimes, primary hemostasis or coagulation disorders.
- Rarely, platelet dysfunctions [11, 12].

Other common abnormal bleeding includes epistaxis, menorrhagia, and gingival bleeding.

Cytopenia

- Cytopenia occurs in all untreated patients with GD1.
- Thrombocytopenia, leukopenia, and anemia can be done simultaneously or independently.
- The pattern of blood cell alteration is dependent on spleen status.
- Thrombocytopenia is caused by hypersplenism, bone marrow involvement, and splenic pooling of platelets.
- Some patients with GD1 suffer from immune thrombocytopenia, which should be considered in individuals with persistent thrombocytopenia despite GD-specific therapy.
- Multiple factors are involved in anemia, such as hypersplenism, B12 or iron deficiency, hemodilution, and decreased erythropoiesis (due to bone marrow infiltration from the Gaucher cell or medullary infarction) [13, 14].

Skeletal Disease

Clinical or radiographic evidence of bone involvement occurs in 70–100% of individuals with GD1, leading to decreased quality of life and immobility in these patients [15, 16]. The exact pathophysiology of bone manifestations is poorly known, but some theories have been reported [18]. The presentation of bone involvement includes

Acute or chronic bone pain.
Fractures.
Osteolytic lesions.
Vertebral compression fractures.
Other fragility fractures associated with low bone mineral density.
Subchondral joint collapse with secondary degenerative arthritis [7, 17].

- **Acute Bone Crisis.**
  The most severe manifestation of bone disease is acute, painful bone crises associated with osteonecrosis (avascular necrosis) with joint collapse in the long bones (proximal and distal femur, proximal tibia, and proximal humerus) and sometimes in the flat bone [7].
  Some mechanisms are proposed for acute bone crisis:
  - The vascular theory is the cornerstone of acute bone pain crises.
  - A mechanical theory has also explained the microfractures (especially on the femoral head or condyle and the tibial plateau).
  - Macrophage-derived mediators [19, 20].
  - Alterations in the bone marrow, immune cells, or cytokine hormones and inflammation.
  - Acute painful bone crises occur more frequently in children (30%).
  - These crises usually develop in 7–10 days, and affected lesions are accompanied by local inflammation, fever, and leukocytosis, like osteomyelitis (pseudo-osteomyelitis), but blood culture is sterile [16, 21].
- **Bone Loss.**
  The prevalence of osteopenia and osteoporosis increases with age, and bone loss occurs earlier and may lead to pathological fractures. Bone mass loss may be associated with other bone and visceral involvement [22].
- **Bone Cyst.**
  Cyst-like lesions in the mandible and the loss of trabecular structure are related to dental abnormalities.
- **Bone Tumor.**
  Secondary bone tumors, including osteosarcoma and osteoblastoma, have been reported [23].
- **Bone Deformity.**
  - During childhood, defects in bone remodeling can result in the enlargement of the metaphyseal and diaphyseal region of the distal part of the femur, called Erlenmeyer flask bone deformity [24].
  - Bone disease in patients with GD1 may not correlate with the severity of hematologic or visceral problems.

Pulmonary Disease

- Interstitial lung disease results in the infiltration of alveolar and interstitial spaces by Gaucher cells.
- Alveolar infiltrations lead to pulmonary fibrosis and restrictive lung disease (secondary to spinal deformation).
- Occlusion of pulmonary capillaries by abnormal cells and soluble mediators in the remodeling of pulmonary vasculature is associated with pulmonary arterial hypertension [25, 26].
- Hepatopulmonary syndrome is caused by the formation of abnormal vascular shunting, which leads to dyspnea, cyanosis with distal finger clubbing, and hypoxemia on standing [8, 27].

Neurological and Psychological Disease

Based on the underlying pathogenesis of the disease, primary central nervous system (CNS) involvement is not expected in GD1, but some neurologic complications remain, including

- Spinal cord or nerve root compression secondary to bone disease (coagulopathy) and peripheral polyneuropathy (14%) [28].

- The association between GD1 and Parkinson's disease (PD).
  - This association was first proposed in 1990 [29].
  - The probability of developing Parkinson's disease (PD) in the general population is nearly 3–4%, while the prevalence of this neurological disorder has been estimated to be higher among other heterozygote members of the family.
  - *GBA1* gene mutations are a genetic risk factor for developing PD up to 5–30 times more than the general population, depending on age, race, and the type of mutation.
  - Approximately, 21% of patients with GD1 may have at least one finding consistent with PD, even if they do not fully have indicators.
  - Five to 15% of people with PD carry a mutation in the *GBA1* gene [30–34].
  - Since PD only occurs in some patients with GD1, other predisposing factors (genetic or environmental) are also involved in developing PD.
  - There is no relationship between the severity of PD and the severity of GD, spleen status, or *GBA1* genotype, but the severity index score in patients with PD/GD1 is higher than GD1 alone [31].
  - The underlying mechanism between PD and GD1 is not entirely known, but the reduction of GCase activity leads to the accumulation of substrates, such as glucosylceramide, glucosylsphingosine, glycosylated cholesterol, and α-synuclein in neurons, particularly in the substantia nigra region. This accumulation results in defects in the function of neurotransmitters, especially dopaminergic.
  - A perturbation of the communication network between three proteins—cathepsin D (important in the degradation of α-synuclein and prosaposin), prosaposin (essential for GCase activity and progranulin transport), and progranulin (effect on lysosome biogenesis, prosaposin trafficking and cathepsin D)—has been explained [35].
  - The clinical manifestations of *GBA*-PD are indistinguishable from sporadic PD, but *GBA*-PD usually occurs at a younger age (on average, 5 years earlier than the sporadic type), and cognitive impairment is greater [34].
  - There are main motor triad symptoms in *GBA*-PD, like the sporadic type, but they can progress rapidly, and nonmotor symptoms are more common and severe in *GBA*-PD [30, 34].
  - Patients with GD have moderate to severe psychological problems, including depressed mood and somatic concerns [36].

Malignancy

- Increased prevalence of hematologic (lymphoma, leukemia, multiple myeloma, non-Hodgkin's lymphoma) and other malignancies (hepatocellular carcinoma, pancreatic cancer) has been reported [37–40].
- The underlying mechanism predisposing to malignancy is unknown, but pathogenic variants in modifier genes may be involved.

Metabolic Abnormalities

- There is increased resting energy expenditure because of elevated cytokine levels and low peripheral insulin and adiponectin level.
- Serum levels of ferritin, chitotriosidase, pulmonary and activation-regulated chemokine (PARC)/C-C motif chemokine ligand 18 (CCL18), angiotensin-converting enzyme, and tartrate-resistant acid phosphatase are usually elevated.
- Insulin resistance and lipid abnormalities (low levels of total and high-density lipoprotein (HDL) cholesterol) have been reported [41, 42].

Immunologic Abnormalities

- Children or adults with GD may have polyclonal gammopathy, but monoclonal gammopathy has only been reported in adult patients [43].

- On the other hand, alterations in cellular immune profiles, such as elevated peripheral blood natural killer T-cell (NKT) lymphocytes and a reduction in normal dendritic cells, may occur [44].

Renal Disease

- Renal disorders, such as proteinuria and hematuria associated with the infiltration of glomeruli by Gaucher cells, have been reported in patients with GD1 [45].

GD Type 2

- An incidence of GD2 from less than 5–20% has been reported [46].
- GD2 is characterized by early, acute, and severe neurological impairment starting before age 2 years, with a rapidly progressive course leading to death by age 2–4 years [1].
- The triad for the diagnosis of this type of GD includes.
  - Pyramidal signs (opisthotonos, head retroflexion, spasticity, and trismus).
  - Bulbar signs (squint, stridor, and swallowing difficulty).
  - Oculomotor paralysis (strabismus, horizontal saccade, and bulbar palsy or paresis)—this is very indicative and a major early sign of the disease [47].
- Apnea associated with severe laryngeal spasms appears later.
- Following this, seizures manifest as generalized tonic-clonic and myoclonic epilepsy, which are often resistant to routine antiepileptic drugs [48].
- Visceral involvement, such as hepatosplenomegaly, is extensive, with severe thrombocytopenia (related to splenomegaly) occurring in 60% of cases [49].
- The downhill clinical course is rapid, with severe spasticity, growth retardation, and cachexia.
- Lung disease results from repeated aspiration, infections, and pulmonary infiltration by Gaucher cells [47].
- The perinatal-lethal form is the rarest and the most severe type of GD. Clinical manifestations of this type of GD begin prenatally or in the neonatal period and include hydrops fetalis (accumulation of fluid in at least two body areas), congenital ichthyosis, and the collodion baby phenotype (a thick and shiny membrane).
- Hepatosplenomegaly, pancytopenia, ichthyosis, arthrogryposis (35–43%), facial dysmorphia, and death in utero or soon after birth may occur [50, 51].

GD Type 3

- Neurological manifestations (such as subacute or chronic neuronopathic disease) are a hallmark of GD3 and may appear during childhood (mean age at onset is 5 years), adolescence, or sometimes adulthood.
- GD3 is clinically heterogeneous, with the mean age of onset of neurological manifestations around 8 years. However, some patients may present before age 2 years with very slow disease progression, with a life expectancy into the third or fourth decade in some patients [52, 53]. Differentiating the latter phenotype is often tricky and can be difficult for GD2, especially in the first 6–9 months of life.
- Neuropathic GD presents as a phenotypic continuum, ranging from horizontal ocular saccades at the mild end of the spectrum to hydrops fetalis at the severe end [1].
- The most common clinical manifestations of GD3 are supranuclear saccadic horizontal gaze palsy associated with severe systemic involvement [48].
- Brain stem auditory evoked response (BAER) testing showed abnormal waveforms (III and IV).
- GD3 is classified into three important forms:
  - **Type 3a**: neurological manifestations of this type are ataxia, progressive dementia, myoclonus, myoclonic seizures, supranuclear gaze palsy, and strabismus. Patients have mild hepatosplenomegaly, and bone disease is variable [54].
  - **Type 3b**: massive hepatosplenomegaly and bone involvement (barreled chest and kyphoscoliosis) associated with mild CNS disorders, including supranuclear gaze

palsy, with or without learning disabilities, have been explained [55].

Electroencephalography reveals generalized background slowing or epileptiform discharges [56]. Most patients do not experience a progressive and degenerative course [55].

The homozygous variant c.1448 T > C allele (p. L483P) in the *GBA1* gene is related to this phenotype. Ophthalmologic manifestations including abnormalities of the retina, cornea, vitreous, uvea, conjunctiva, and eye movements have been recognized [57, 58].

Some patients have intelligence quotients (IQs) below the mean, along with learning and functional disabilities, while others may have above-average IQs [56].

The verbal IQ is higher than the performance IQ, which may be related to visual-spatial deficits caused by eye movement abnormalities [59].

- **Type 3c or cardiovascular form**: this type of GD3 is rare and characterized by cardiovascular calcification, corneal opacity, supranuclear gaze palsy, and noncommunicating hydrocephalus. There is a mild visceral and bone involvement [60].

Cardiac involvement (heart valve and aortic calcification), mild hepatosplenomegaly, supranuclear gaze palsy, and bone involvement are associated with homozygosity for the D409H mutation in the *GBA1* gene. Neurological manifestations can appear later, and progression is variable [61].

3.3 Comorbidities Associated with Gaucher Disease

There are some comorbidities associated with GD, including

- Celiac disease.
- Hashimoto thyroiditis.
- Immune thrombocytopenia.

These diseases should be considered if symptoms of GD (for example, growth retardation, pancytopenia) do not respond well to enzyme replacement therapy (ERT) [62]. A summary of clinical symptoms of GD1 at different ages is shown in Table 3.1.

Table 3.1 Clinical manifestations of GD

Age	Prenatal	Infancy	Childhood	Adolescence
Clinical manifestations	Congenital ichthyosis	Hepatosplenomegaly	Hepatosplenomegaly	Hepatosplenomegaly
	Collodion baby	Thrombocytopenia	Pancytopenia	Pancytopenia
	Hepatosplenomegaly	Seizures	Bleeding tendency	Bleeding tendency
	Pancytopenia	Pyramidal signs	Bone involvement	Bone crisis
	Ichthyosis	Laryngeal spasms	Saccadic horizontal	Osteoporosis
	Arthrogryposis	Failure to thrive	Gaze palsy	Delay of puberty
	Facial dysmorphia	Cardiac valve calcification	Strabismus	Pulmonary infiltration
	Death	Corneal opacity	Neurological involvement	
		Supranuclear gaze palsy		
		Bulbar signs		

3.4 Pathologic Findings in GD

- The cornerstone of GD is Gaucher cells (macrophages laden with lipids), with wrinkled tissue paper being their characteristic histologic feature. Electron microscopy reveals cytoplasmic inclusions that are tubular or spindle shaped with diameters ranging from 0.6 to 4 μm, containing many small tubules measuring 13–75 nm in diameter [63].
- Neuropathologic examination shows the involvement of the globus pallidus, caudate, frontal cortex, pons, thalamus, and cerebellum in patients with GD2. The most common changes include gliosis, periadventitial Gaucher cells, free Gaucher cells, neuronal loss, and neuronophagia. These findings may be due to the accumulation of neurotoxic substrates such as glycolipid and glucosylsphingosine [64, 65].

3.5 Radiologic Investigations

Imaging studies can suggest the diagnosis of GD and/or its complications.

- **Bone Magnetic Resonance Imaging (MRI).**
  - This method is preferred for evaluating bone involvement in GD.
  - T1-weighted sequences can detect bone marrow infiltration, while T2-weighted sequences are considered for the assessment of bone complications such as infarction or avascular necrosis [66].
  - MRI can be used to assess the extent of lesions and the presence of recent complications.
  - Quantitative chemical shift imaging MRI is used for semi-quantitative bone marrow infiltration, which mostly occurs at the proximal and distal ends.
  - Hypointense signals in T1-weighted sequences reflect the replacement of normal bone marrow fat by Gaucher cells.
  - Evaluation of bone marrow involvement is more difficult in younger patients because of the presence of red bone marrow in the long bones [67].
  - Whole-body MRI is used for disease monitoring.
- **X-ray Image**s.
  - Erlenmeyer flask deformity caused by the abnormal remodeling of the metaphysis in the lower third of the femurs is detected by bone radiographs (Fig. 3.2).
  - Other defects found by X-ray include bone infarct sequelae, avascular necrosis, thinning of the cortical bone, lytic lesions, and the sequelae of traumatic and pathological fractures [68]. The sensitivity of standard radiological imaging for the detection of bone defects in GD is poor and not recommended for monitoring due to the risk or radiation exposure [66].
- **Bone Mineral Densitometry (BMD).**
  - BMD lumbar spine and femoral regions are used to diagnose osteopenia or osteoporosis in adults and children >5 years old.
  - According to recent guidelines, osteopenia is defined as a T score between −1 and −2.5 and osteoporosis as a T score ≤ −2.5.

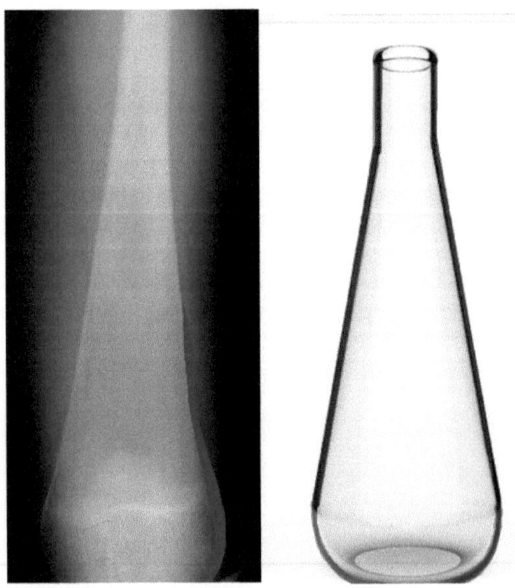

Fig. 3.2 Erlenmeyer flask deformity picture in a patient with GD1

  - The severity of osteopenia in patients with GD correlates with genotype, the severity of splenomegaly, and hepatomegaly [22].
- **Bone Scintigraphy.**
  - ^{99m}Tc bone scintigraphy is used to diagnose the possibility of a bone lesion if MRI is not available. Indeed, clinically asymptomatic bone lesions or sequelae, especially in atypical sites (jaws, feet, hands), and fractures can be detected by scintigraphy.
- **Abdominal Imaging.**
  - Abdominal magnetic resonance imaging (MRI) is the preferable method for assessing liver and spleen diameter/volume and morphology. But abdominal ultrasound may be used if MRI is unavailable or in cases of uncontrollable claustrophobia.
  - Computed tomography (CT) has previously been used for estimating Gaucher organ volumes, but because of justifiable concerns about CT radiation, MRI is preferred [68].

3.6 Differential Diagnosis of GD

- **Saposin C deficiency or prosaposin deficiency**: saposin C acts as a cofactor for the glucocerebrosidase enzyme. Pathogenic variants in the *PSAP* gene lead to saposin C deficiency, which presents with symptoms like severe neuropathic or nonneuronopathic GD. These patients have normal glucocerebrosidase enzyme activity [69, 70]. In fact, saposin C has multiple roles in glycosphingolipid (GSL) catabolism and CNS function, especially in axonal integrity independent of its role as a stabilizer of GCase.
- Gaucher-like cells may be found in other storage disorders, such as Niemann-Pick disease type C. Some clinical presentations, such as ataxia, supranuclear gaze palsy, pseudobulbar signs, and splenomegaly, are compatible with both GD type 3 and NP-C. In contrast to Gaucher disease, which exhibits horizontal supranuclear gaze palsy, Niemann-Pick type C shows vertical supranuclear gaze palsy.
- Sometimes, pseudo-Gaucher cells have been shown in some hematologic diseases, including myeloproliferative and myelodysplastic disorders [71].
- Osteonecrosis, like GD, may occur in an individual with Legg-Calvé-Perthes disease (LCPD). LCPD is caused by a pathogenic mutation in the *COL2A1* gene, which is inherited in an autosomal dominant pattern [72].
- Ichthyosis and collodion skin are also reported in congenital ichthyosis [73].
- Hydrops fetalis is observed in other lysosomal storage diseases, including sialidosis type 1, GM1 gangliosidosis, mucopolysaccharidosis types VII and IV, Wolman disease, Niemann-Pick disease type C, mucolipidosis II, galactosialidosis, Farber disease, and free sialic acid storage disease [74].
- Erlenmeyer flask deformity has been described in some disorders, including fibrous dysplasia, osteopetrosis, Niemann-Pick disease, and heavy metal poisoning [68].

Learning Points

- Gaucher disease presents in various forms and should be considered in any patient with unexplained splenomegaly, hematological, skeletal, or neurological symptoms.
- There is an overlap among and within the forms of GD, indicating that GD is a continuum of manifestations rather than three distinct subtypes.
- GD1 is differentiated from GD2 (acute neuropathic) and GD3 (chronic neuropathic) by the lack of neurologic involvement.
- GD1 is defined by the lack of neurological symptoms and accounts for about 90% of all cases of GD. It can be present at any age.
- GD2 is characterized by early, acute, and severe neurological impairment starting before age 2 years, with a rapidly progressive course.
- Neurological manifestations (as subacute or chronic neuronopathic disease) are a hallmark of GD3 and may appear during childhood (mean age at onset is 5 years), adolescence, or sometimes adulthood.

References

1. Goker-Alpan O, Schiffmann R, Park JK, Stubblefield BK, Tayebi N, Sidransky E. Phenotypic continuum in neuronopathic Gaucher disease: an intermediate phenotype between type 2 and type 3. J Pediatr. 2003;143(2):273–6.
2. Sidransky E. Gaucher disease: complexity in a "simple" disorder. Mol Genet Metab. 2004;83(1–2):6–15.
3. Charrow J, Andersson HC, Kaplan P, Kolodny EH, Mistry P, Pastores G, et al. The Gaucher registry: demographics and disease characteristics of 1698 patients with Gaucher disease. Arch Intern Med. 2000;160(18):2835–43.
4. Elstein D, Gellman A, Altarescu G, Abrahamov A, Hadas-Halpern I, Phillips M, et al. Disease severity in sibling pairs with type 1 Gaucher disease. J Inherit Metab Dis. 2010;33(1):79–83.
5. Kaplan P, Andersson HC, Kacena KA, Yee JD. The clinical and demographic characteristics of nonneuronopathic Gaucher disease in 887 children at diagnosis. Arch Pediatr Adolesc Med. 2006;160(6):603–8.
6. Elstein D, Abrahamov A, Dweck A, Hadas-Halpern I, Zimran A. Gaucher disease: pediatric concerns. Paediatr Drugs. 2002;4(7):417–26.
7. Grabowski GA, Andria G, Baldellou A, Campbell PE, Charrow J, Cohen IJ, et al. Pediatric non-neuronopathic Gaucher disease: presentation, diagnosis and assessment. Consensus statements. Eur J Pediatr. 2004;163(2):58–66.
8. Lachmann RH, Wight DG, Lomas DJ, Fisher NC, Schofield JP, Elias E, et al. Massive hepatic fibrosis in Gaucher's disease: clinico-pathological and radiological features. QJM. 2000;93(4):237–44.
9. Regenboog M, Bohte AE, Somers I, van Delden OM, Maas M, Hollak CE. Imaging characteristics of focal splenic and hepatic lesions in type 1 Gaucher disease. Blood Cells Mol Dis. 2016;60:49–57.
10. Taddei TH, Dziura J, Chen S, Yang R, Hyogo H, Sullards C, et al. High incidence of cholesterol gallstone disease in type 1 Gaucher disease: characterizing the biliary phenotype of type 1 Gaucher disease. J Inherit Metab Dis. 2010;33(3):291–300.
11. Gillis S, Hyam E, Abrahamov A, Elstein D, Zimran A. Platelet function abnormalities in Gaucher disease patients. Am J Hematol. 1999;61(2):103–6.
12. Rosenbaum H. Hemorrhagic aspects of Gaucher disease. Rambam Maimonides Med J. 2014;5(4):e0039.
13. Thomas AS, Mehta AB, Hughes DA. Diagnosing Gaucher disease: an on-going need for increased awareness amongst haematologists. Blood Cells Mol Dis. 2013;50(3):212–7.
14. Zimran A, Gelbart T, Beutler E. Linkage of the PvuII polymorphism with the common Jewish mutation for Gaucher disease. Am J Hum Genet. 1990;46(5):902–5.
15. Baldellou A, Andria G, Campbell PE, Charrow J, Cohen IJ, Grabowski GA, et al. Paediatric non-neuronopathic Gaucher disease: recommendations for treatment and monitoring. Eur J Pediatr. 2004;163(2):67–75.
16. Wenstrup RJ, Roca-Espiau M, Weinreb NJ, Bembi B. Skeletal aspects of Gaucher disease: a review. Br J Radiol. 2002;75(Suppl 1):A2–12.
17. Pastores GM, Patel MJ, Firooznia H. Bone and joint complications related to Gaucher disease. Curr Rheumatol Rep. 2000;2(2):175–80.
18. Reed M, Baker RJ, Mehta AB, Hughes DA. Enhanced differentiation of osteoclasts from mononuclear precursors in patients with Gaucher disease. Blood Cells Mol Dis. 2013;51(3):185–94.
19. Clarke LA, Hollak CE. The clinical spectrum and pathophysiology of skeletal complications in lysosomal storage disorders. Best Pract Res Clin Endocrinol Metab. 2015;29(2):219–35.
20. Marcucci G, Zimran A, Bembi B, Kanis J, Reginster JY, Rizzoli R, et al. Gaucher disease and bone manifestations. Calcif Tissue Int. 2014;95(6):477–94.
21. Pastores GM, Meere PA. Musculoskeletal complications associated with lysosomal storage disorders: Gaucher disease and hurler-Scheie syndrome (muco-

polysaccharidosis type I). Curr Opin Rheumatol. 2005;17(1):70–8.
22. Pastores GM, Wallenstein S, Desnick RJ, Luckey MM. Bone density in type 1 Gaucher disease. J Bone Miner Res. 1996;11(11):1801–7.
23. Zver S, Bracko M, Andoljsek D. Primary bone angiosarcoma in a patient with Gaucher disease. Int J Hematol. 2010;92(2):374–7.
24. Bembi B, Ciana G, Mengel E, Terk MR, Martini C, Wenstrup RJ. Bone complications in children with Gaucher disease. Br J Radiol. 2002;75(Suppl 1):A37–44.
25. Elstein D, Nir A, Klutstein M, Rudensky B, Zimran A. C-reactive protein and NT-proBNP as surrogate markers for pulmonary hypertension in Gaucher disease. Blood Cells Mol Dis. 2005;34(3):201–5.
26. Ross DJ, Spira S, Buchbinder NA. Gaucher cells in pulmonary-capillary blood in association with pulmonary hypertension. N Engl J Med. 1997;336(5):379–81.
27. Miller A, Brown LK, Pastores GM, Desnick RJ. Pulmonary involvement in type 1 Gaucher disease: functional and exercise findings in patients with and without clinical interstitial lung disease. Clin Genet. 2003;63(5):368–76.
28. Biegstraaten M, Mengel E, Maródi L, Petakov M, Niederau C, Giraldo P, et al. Peripheral neuropathy in adult type 1 Gaucher disease: a 2-year prospective observational study. Brain. 2010;133(10):2909–19.
29. Tayebi N, Callahan M, Madike V, Stubblefield BK, Orvisky E, Krasnewich D, et al. Gaucher disease and parkinsonism: a phenotypic and genotypic characterization. Mol Genet Metab. 2001;73(4):313–21.
30. Alcalay RN, Dinur T, Quinn T, Sakanaka K, Levy O, Waters C, et al. Comparison of Parkinson risk in Ashkenazi Jewish patients with Gaucher disease and GBA heterozygotes. JAMA Neurol. 2014;71(6):752–7.
31. Bultron G, Kacena K, Pearson D, Boxer M, Yang R, Sathe S, et al. The risk of Parkinson's disease in type 1 Gaucher disease. J Inherit Metab Dis. 2010;33(2):167–73.
32. Gan-Or Z, Amshalom I, Kilarski LL, Bar-Shira A, Gana-Weisz M, Mirelman A, et al. Differential effects of severe vs mild GBA mutations on Parkinson disease. Neurology. 2015;84(9):880–7.
33. Neumann J, Bras J, Deas E, O'Sullivan SS, Parkkinen L, Lachmann RH, et al. Glucocerebrosidase mutations in clinical and pathologically proven Parkinson's disease. Brain. 2009;132(Pt 7):1783–94.
34. Sidransky E, Nalls MA, Aasly JO, Aharon-Peretz J, Annesi G, Barbosa ER, et al. Multicenter analysis of glucocerebrosidase mutations in Parkinson's disease. N Engl J Med. 2009;361(17):1651–61.
35. Tayebi N, Lopez G, Do J, Sidransky E, Pro-cathepsin D. Prosaposin, and progranulin: lysosomal networks in parkinsonism. Trends Mol Med. 2020;26(10):913–23.
36. Packman W, Wilson Crosbie T, Riesner A, Fairley C, Packman S. Psychological complications of patients with Gaucher disease. J Inherit Metab Dis. 2006;29(1):99–105.
37. Kojiro M, Kage M, Abe H, Imamura M, Shiraishi K, Mizoguchi M. Association of dysgerminoma and Gaucher's disease. Cancer. 1983;51(4):712–5.
38. Landgren O, Turesson I, Gridley G, Caporaso NE. Risk of malignant disease among 1525 adult male US veterans with Gaucher disease. Arch Intern Med. 2007;167(11):1189–94.
39. Lo SM, Stein P, Mullaly S, Bar M, Jain D, Pastores GM, et al. Expanding spectrum of the association between type 1 Gaucher disease and cancers: a series of patients with up to 3 sequential cancers of multiple types – correlation with genotype and phenotype. Am J Hematol. 2010;85(5):340–5.
40. Madeo A, Garaventa A, Sementa AR, Suffia C, Di Rocco M. The unusual association between neuroblastoma and Gaucher disease: case report and review of the literature. Blood Cells Mol Dis. 2018;68:106–8.
41. de Fost M, Langeveld M, Franssen R, Hutten BA, Groener JE, de Groot E, et al. Low HDL cholesterol levels in type I Gaucher disease do not lead to an increased risk of cardiovascular disease. Atherosclerosis. 2009;204(1):267–72.
42. Langeveld M, de Fost M, Aerts JM, Sauerwein HP, Hollak CE. Overweight, insulin resistance and type II diabetes in type I Gaucher disease patients in relation to enzyme replacement therapy. Blood Cells Mol Dis. 2008;40(3):428–32.
43. Wine E, Yaniv I, Cohen IJ. Hyperimmunoglobulinemia in pediatric-onset type 1 Gaucher disease and effects of enzyme replacement therapy. J Pediatr Hematol Oncol. 2007;29(7):451–7.
44. Micheva I, Marinakis T, Repa C, Kouraklis-Symeonidis A, Vlacha V, Anagnostopoulos N, et al. Dendritic cells in patients with type I Gaucher disease are decreased in number but functionally normal. Blood Cells Mol Dis. 2006;36(2):298–307.
45. Santoro D, Rosenbloom BE, Cohen AH. Gaucher disease with nephrotic syndrome: response to enzyme replacement therapy. Am J Kidney Dis. 2002;40(1):E4.
46. Tajima A, Yokoi T, Ariga M, Ito T, Kaneshiro E, Eto Y, et al. Clinical and genetic study of Japanese patients with type 3 Gaucher disease. Mol Genet Metab. 2009;97(4):272–7.
47. Mignot C, Doummar D, Maire I, De Villemeur TB. Type 2 Gaucher disease: 15 new cases and review of the literature. Brain Dev. 2006;28(1):39–48.
48. Roshan Lal T, Sidransky E. The Spectrum of neurological manifestations associated with Gaucher disease. Diseases. 2017;5(1)
49. Finn LS, Zhang M, Chen SH, Scott CR. Severe type II Gaucher disease with ichthyosis, arthrogryposis and neuronal apoptosis: molecular and pathological analyses. Am J Med Genet. 2000;91(3):222–6.
50. Carr PC, Casamiquela KM, Jacks SK. Gaucher disease type 2 presenting with collodion membrane and blueberry muffin lesions. Pediatr Dermatol. 2016;33(1):e20–2.
51. Mignot C, Gelot A, Bessières B, Daffos F, Voyer M, Menez F, et al. Perinatal-lethal Gaucher disease. Am J Med Genet A. 2003;120a(3):338–44.

52. Stirnemann J, Belmatoug N, Camou F, Serratrice C, Froissart R, Caillaud C, et al. A review of Gaucher disease pathophysiology, clinical presentation and treatments. Int J Mol Sci. 2017;18(2)
53. Tylki-Szymańska A, Vellodi A, El-Beshlawy A, Cole JA, Kolodny E. Neuronopathic Gaucher disease: demographic and clinical features of 131 patients enrolled in the international collaborative Gaucher group neurological outcomes subregistry. J Inherit Metab Dis. 2010;33(4):339–46.
54. Cox TM, Schofield JP. Gaucher's disease: clinical features and natural history. Baillieres Clin Haematol. 1997;10(4):657–89.
55. Steward AM, Wiggs E, Lindstrom T, Ukwuani S, Ryan E, Tayebi N, et al. Variation in cognitive function over time in Gaucher disease type 3. Neurology. 2019;93(24):e2272–e83.
56. Benko W, Ries M, Wiggs EA, Brady RO, Schiffmann R, Fitzgibbon EJ. The saccadic and neurological deficits in type 3 Gaucher disease. PLoS One. 2011;6(7):e22410.
57. Donald A, Tan CY, Chakrapani A, Hughes DA, Sharma R, Cole D, et al. Eye movement biomarkers allow for the definition of phenotypes in Gaucher disease. Orphanet J Rare Dis. 2020;15(1):349.
58. Eghbali A, Hassan S, Seehra G, FitzGibbon E, Sidransky E. Ophthalmological findings in Gaucher disease. Mol Genet Metab. 2019;127(1):23–7.
59. Altarescu G, Hill S, Wiggs E, Jeffries N, Kreps C, Parker CC, et al. The efficacy of enzyme replacement therapy in patients with chronic neuronopathic Gaucher's disease. J Pediatr. 2001;138(4):539–47.
60. Kurolap A, Del Toro M, Spiegel R, Gutstein A, Shafir G, Cohen IJ, et al. Gaucher disease type 3c: new patients with unique presentations and review of the literature. Mol Genet Metab. 2019;127(2):138–46.
61. Michelakakis H, Skardoutsou A, Mathioudakis J, Moraitou M, Dimitriou E, Voudris C, et al. Early-onset severe neurological involvement and D409H homozygosity in Gaucher disease: outcome of enzyme replacement therapy. Blood Cells Mol Dis. 2002;28(1):1–4.
62. González DC, Ruiz A, Oliveri B. Osteomalacia as an extraintestinal manifestation of Celiac disease in a patient treated for Gaucher disease. Endocr Metab Sci. 2020;1(1):100052.
63. Beutler E. Monocyte and macrophage disorders: lipid storage disease. In: Williams WJBE, Erslev AJ, Lichman MA, editors. Hematology. New York: McGraw-Hill; 1990.
64. Orvisky E, Park JK, LaMarca ME, Ginns EI, Martin BM, Tayebi N, et al. Glucosylsphingosine accumulation in tissues from patients with Gaucher disease: correlation with phenotype and genotype. Mol Genet Metab. 2002;76(4):262–70.
65. Wong K, Sidransky E, Verma A, Mixon T, Sandberg GD, Wakefield LK, et al. Neuropathology provides clues to the pathophysiology of Gaucher disease. Mol Genet Metab. 2004;82(3):192–207.
66. Vom Dahl S, Poll L, Di Rocco M, Ciana G, Denes C, Mariani G, et al. Evidence-based recommendations for monitoring bone disease and the response to enzyme replacement therapy in Gaucher patients. Curr Med Res Opin. 2006;22(6):1045–64.
67. Hollak C, Maas M, Akkerman E, den Heeten A, Aerts H. Dixon quantitative chemical shift imaging is a sensitive tool for the evaluation of bone marrow responses to individualized doses of enzyme supplementation therapy in type 1 Gaucher disease. Blood Cells Mol Dis. 2001;27(6):1005–12.
68. Maas M, Poll LW, Terk MR. Imaging and quantifying skeletal involvement in Gaucher disease. Br J Radiol. 2002;75(Suppl 1):A13–24.
69. Qi X, Grabowski GA. Molecular and cell biology of acid beta-glucosidase and prosaposin. Prog Nucleic Acid Res Mol Biol. 2001;66:203–39.
70. Tylki-Szymańska A, Czartoryska B, Vanier MT, Poorthuis BJ, Groener JA, Ługowska A, et al. Non-neuronopathic Gaucher disease due to Saposin C deficiency. Clin Genet. 2007;72(6):538–42.
71. Stewart AJ, Jones RD. Pseudo-Gaucher cells in myelodysplasia. J Clin Pathol. 1999;52(12):917–8.
72. Kenet G, Hayek S, Mor M, Lubetsky A, Miller L, Rosenberg N, et al. The 1226G (N370S) Gaucher mutation among patients with Legg-Calve-Perthes disease. Blood Cells Mol Dis. 2003;31(1):72–4.
73. Srivastava P, Srivastava A, Srivastava P, Betigeri AV, Verma M. Congenital ichthyosis—collodion baby case report. J Clin Diagn Res. 2016;10(6):Sj01-2.
74. Kooper AJ, Janssens PM, de Groot AN, Liebrand-van Sambeek ML, van den Berg CJ, Tan-Sindhunata GB, et al. Lysosomal storage diseases in non-immune hydrops fetalis pregnancies. Clin Chim Acta. 2006;371(1–2):176–82.

4 Overview of Diagnostic Approach to Gaucher Disease

Ali Talea, Mahsa Mohammad Amoli, and Parastoo Rostami

4.1 Introduction

Diagnosis of GD is often delayed several years after the onset of the first clinical and laboratory presentation due to a lack of awareness of the disease and the challenges in both biochemical and genetic diagnosis of GD (Fig. 4.1).

Some patients with GD are identified after bone marrow aspiration for evaluation of thrombocytopenia, splenomegaly, and chronic anemia or after liver biopsy because of hepatomegaly, and then Gaucher cells are found.

Since Gaucher disease is common in Ashkenazi-origin individuals, Mistry et al. introduced two algorithms for the diagnostic approach to Ashkenazi and non-Ashkenazi populations (Fig. 4.2). Confirming the diagnosis of Gaucher disease in a patient who suspected of GD should be based on the assessment of glucocerebrosidase activity and molecular studies [1]. Diagnostic approach to GD includes the following.

4.2 Enzyme Activity Assay

The gold standard for diagnosing Gaucher disease is the β-glucocerebrosidase (BGLU) enzyme activity assay in blood leucocytes and cultured skin fibroblasts, where the enzyme drops below 10% of the normal level [2].

Enzyme activity varies among peripheral leukocytes, cultured skin fibroblasts, and other mononuclear cells, with β-glucocerebrosidase function decreasing from monocytes to lymphocytes to granulocytes [3–5].

BGLU activity is assessed using artificial substrates through fluorometric methods, tandem mass spectrometry, or digital microfluidics. The fluorometric method is the gold standard for leukocyte and fibroblast lysates, while tandem mass spectrometry and digital microfluidics are typically employed for screening studies involving dried blood spot (DBS) samples [6].

The 4-methylumbelliferyl-beta-glucoside assay shows that GD1 patients retain residual enzymatic activity (10–15% of normal), while GD2 and GD3 patients exhibit similar lower enzyme activity. Additionally, acid β-glucosidase activity may appear falsely low in cases of saposin deficiency, mutant enzyme trafficking defects,

A. Talea
Molecular-Cellular Endocrinology and Metabolism Research Institute, Tehran University of Medical Sciences (TUMS), Tehran, Iran

M. M. Amoli
Medical Genetics, Metabolic Disorders Research Center, Endocrinology and Metabolism Molecular-Cellular Sciences Institute, Tehran University of Medical Sciences, Tehran, Iran
e-mail: amolimm@tums.ac.ir

P. Rostami (✉)
Research Center for Growth and Development, Division of Endocrinology and Metabolism, Department of Pediatrics, Pediatrics Center of Excellence, Tehran University of Medical Sciences, Tehran, Iran

© The Author(s), under exclusive license to Springer Nature Singapore Pte Ltd. 2025

P. Rostami, A. Talea (eds.), *Gaucher Disease*, https://doi.org/10.1007/978-981-96-4763-7_4

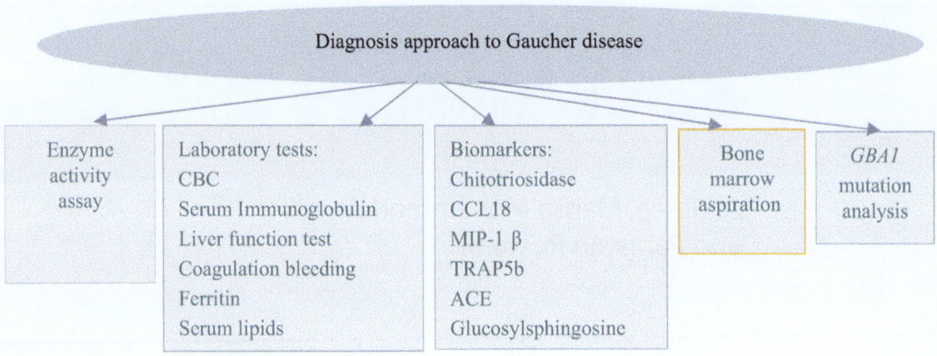

Fig. 4.1 Diagnostic approach to GD

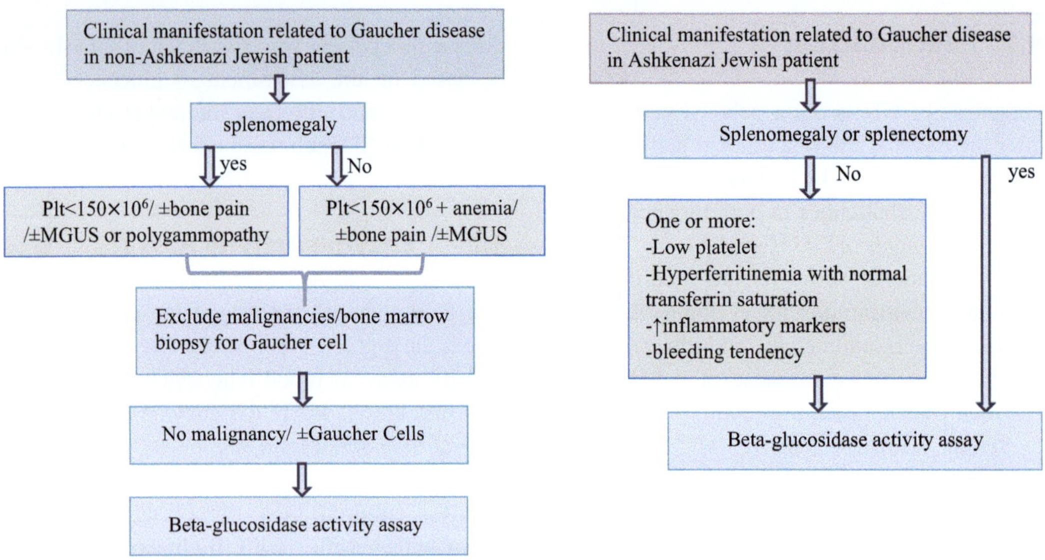

Fig. 4.2 Diagnosis algorithm for Ashkenazi (right) and non-Ashkenazi (left) individuals suspected of Gaucher disease type 1. *MGUS* monoclonal gammopathy of undetermined significance [63]

or other lysosomal storage disorders, such as Niemann-Pick type C disease (Fig. 4.3). In these situations, enzyme activity assay in the cultured skin fibroblasts should be considered [7].

Enzyme activity in DBS samples can serve as a screening test for clinically suspected individuals. BGLU activity below the cut-off values should be verified by measuring BGLU activity in leukocytes or fibroblasts (Fig. 4.4).

Enzyme activity in heterozygous carriers and normal individuals overlaps significantly, making enzyme function assays inadequate for distinguishing between carriers and noncarriers or heterozygous carriers and the normal population [8].

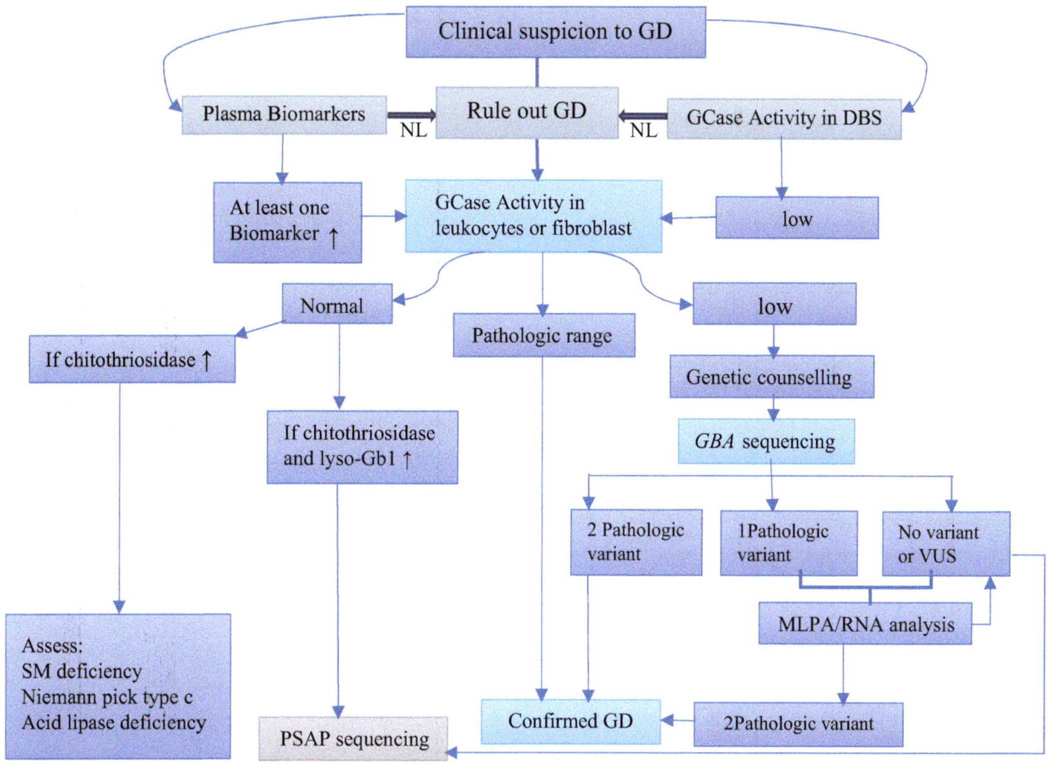

Fig. 4.3 Diagnostic algorithm of GD based on laboratory findings. *SM* sphingomyelinase, *RNA* ribonucleic acid, *MLPA* multiplex ligation-dependent probe amplification, *VUS* variant of uncertain significance [6]

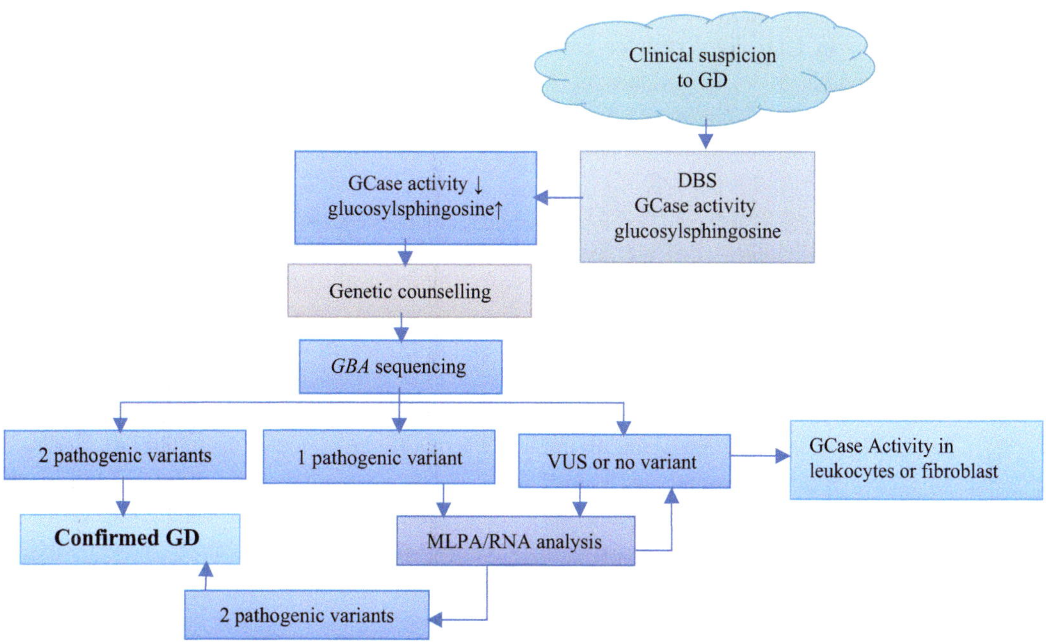

Fig. 4.4 Approach to a patient who is suspected of GD with normal GCase activity in DBS [6]

4.3 Biochemical Tests

There are some biochemical tests used for the investigation of GD in suspected individuals:

- Hemogram tests.
- Hemostasis tests.
- Serum immunoglobulin assay.
- Disease biomarkers.
  - Chitotriosidase.
  - CCL18.
  - Glucosylsphingosine (GlcSph).
  - MIP-1β.
  - TRAP5b and ACE.
  - gpNMB (glycoprotein nonmetastatic melanoma protein B),
  - Other routine blood tests.

4.3.1 Hemogram Tests

- **Hemoglobin levels**: anemia is less common in GD1, and hemoglobin levels rarely decrease to less than 9 g/dl. Different factors are involved in anemia [9].
- **Platelet count**: thrombocytopenia is the most frequent hematologic manifestation of GD1 (90% of cases) in GD1, and platelet count vary from less than 60×10^9 platelets/L to $<120 \times 10^9$ platelets/L. Leukopenia is rare. Blood cell counts may be normal in patients with a history of splenectomy [10].
- Liver enzymes may be mildly elevated [11].
- **Ferritin level**: ferritinemia is common in GD1 and is associated with increased liver volume. Transferrin saturation, serum iron, and soluble transferrin receptor concentrations remain normal [12]. Iron accumulates in the liver and bone marrow during the development of GD. Ferritin levels can be predictive of the onset of bone complications and can be used as a nonspecific marker for monitoring GD [13].

4.3.2 Hemostasis

- Some coagulation abnormalities have been reported in GD, making patients prone to bleeding.
- Factor XI deficiency should be considered in Ashkenazim patients with bleeding [14].

4.3.3 Serum Immunoglobulin

- Polyclonal hypergammaglobulinemia and monoclonal gammopathy are rare conditions in GD1 [15].

4.3.4 Biomarkers

- **Chitotriosidase.**

  Chitotriosidase is an enzyme released by lipid-laden macrophages and is elevated in the plasma of GD patients.

  Serum chitotriosidase levels are directly linked to disease severity and have been used for over 20 years to monitor treatment [16].

  Plasma chitotriosidase activity assay (by 4-methylumbelliferylβ-D-N, N′, N″-triacetyl-chitotrioside (4MU-C3), or 4-methylumbelliferyl deoxychitobiose (4MU-dC2)) is commonly used as a first-line screening test in many centers.

  Chitotriosidase activity in plasma is up to 1000 times higher than the average values in the healthy population.

  Generally, plasma chitotriosidase activity is higher in GD1 than in GD2 and GD3 [17] but also increases in asymptomatic patients and can be used to screen other family members of the patient with GD1.

  The interpretation of plasma chitotriosidase activity can be challenging due to a 24-base pair duplication in the CHIT1 gene, which inhibits the synthesis of the chitotriosidase protein [18].

Elevated plasma chitotriosidase activity is not limited to GD patients. A mild increase in chitotriosidase activity has been observed in various lysosomal and nonlysosomal disorders, including Niemann-Pick type C, congenital herpes virus infection leading to hydrops fetalis, and multiple sclerosis.

Chitotriosidase activity is elevated in the previously mentioned disorders, but it remains lower than in GD, where a significant increase in plasma chitotriosidase activity is both a characteristic and diagnostic marker [16, 17, 19].

- **CCL18.**

  CCL18 (chemokine (C-C motif) ligand 18)/PARC (pulmonary and activation-regulated chemokine) is a member of the C-C chemokine family.

  CCL18/PARC, together with many other macrophage inflammatory proteins (MIPs), is located on chromosome 17 and produced by antigen-presenting cells of the innate immune system, including macrophages, dendritic cells, and monocytes [20].

  Gaucher cells can produce CCL18 and appear at high levels in serum (10–50 times higher than those of controls) but less than the level of chitotriosidase.

  Elevated CCL18 levels, like chitotriosidase, are linked to poorer prognosis. Thus, evaluating CCL18/PARC (through enzyme-linked immunosorbent assay (ELISA) and dissociation-enhanced lanthanide fluoroimmunoassay (DELFIA)) may serve as an alternative biomarker for therapeutic monitoring, especially in patients with chitotriosidase deficiency (Fig. 4.3) [21, 22].

  Patients with alpha-mannosidosis and Niemann-Pick types A and B disease have shown an increase in this biomarker to levels equivalent to those in GD [23].

  Increased PARC/CCL18 levels are found in nonlysosomal storage diseases such as atherosclerosis, rheumatoid arthritis, beta-thalassemia, and sarcoidosis [24].

- **Glucosylsphingosine (GlcSph).**

  Glucosylsphingosine (lyso-Gb1 or lyso-GL1), measured by LC–MS/MS, is a novel biomarker for diagnosing and monitoring Gaucher disease, exhibiting 100% sensitivity and specificity [25, 26].

  In symptomatic GD1, GlcSph levels in plasma increase approximately 180-fold compared to a healthy population [27].

  Mildly elevated plasma GlcSph levels may occur in patients with action myoclonus renal failure syndrome, Niemann-Pick disease type C, and sap C deficiency due to defective LIMP-2 [28–30].

  Chitotriosidase activity, CCL18, and lyso-Gb1 are generally recommended as initial tests for diagnosing GD [6, 31].

  If chitotriosidase activity is normal, a 24 bp duplication in CHIT1 should be excluded. A suspected diagnosis of GD must be confirmed through a GCase activity assay in peripheral blood leukocytes or cultured fibroblast extracts, along with the molecular analysis of the GBA1 gene [6] (Fig. 4.3).

- **MIP-1β.**

  Macrophage inflammatory protein 1β (MIP-1β or CCL4) is also used as a skeletal biomarker in GD.

  Plasma MIP-1β is a biomarker for monitoring skeletal lesions in multiple myeloma, and serum MIP-1β levels increase in patients with GD and bone involvement [32]. MIP-1β levels are expected to decrease during ERT.

- **TRAP5b and ACE.**

  The oldest biomarkers of GD include tartrate-resistant acid phosphatase 5b (TRAP5b) (a biomarker secreted by osteoclasts activity) and angiotensin converting enzyme (ACE), which are not used due to poor specificity [33, 34].

- **gpNMB (Glycoprotein Nonmetastatic Melanoma Protein B),**

  gpNMB is selectively expressed by Gaucher cells and is found in plasma at levels over 50 times higher in patients with GD1. This biomarker has also been identified in Niemann-Pick disease type C. Thus, more studies are needed to use it as a diagnostic biomarker for Gaucher disease [35].

4.3.5 Other Routine Blood Tests

Liver transaminases, bilirubin (both free and conjugated), gamma-glutamyl transferase (GGT), and alkaline phosphatase are not routinely measured, except under certain conditions.

C-reactive protein (CRP) is an inflammatory protein whose levels rise during bone crises or infections, such as cholecystitis [22].

Serum levels of bone formation markers, like osteocalcin, may be low, while bone resorption markers, such as C-telopeptide pyridinoline crosslinks of type-I collagen (ICTP), can be normal to high [36].

GD1 patients show decreased high-density lipoprotein (HDL) cholesterol and ApoA1 levels, with potentially increased triglycerides.

There is no significant difference in carotid intima-media thickness between GD patients and the general population [37].

Screening for polyclonal hypergammaglobulinemia and rare monoclonal gammopathy is recommended [38]. Unlike monoclonal gammopathy, ERT may help reduce polyclonal hypergammaglobulinemia [39].

4.4 Bone Marrow Aspiration (BMA)

- Gaucher disease diagnosis relies on genetic or enzyme activity testing rather than bone marrow aspiration, when cytopenia and hepatomegaly/or splenomegaly are present.
- BMA may be indicated for isolated thrombocytopenia, splenomegaly, and the investigation of coexisting hematologic malignancies, particularly when Gaucher cells are present.
- Distinguishing Gaucher cells from "pseudo-Gaucher" cells, seen in disorders such as human immunodeficiency virus (HIV), thalassemia, mycobacterial infections in immunodeficient patients, and hematological malignancies, is crucial [22, 40].

4.5 *GBA1* Mutation Analysis

Genetic testing is used for several purposes in GD, including the following:

- **Confirmation of Disease Diagnosis.**
  - Diagnosis of Mendelian disorders, including lysosomal storage disorders, typically begins with deoxyribonucleic acid (DNA) sequencing to identify common biallelic pathogenic variants (prior to the enzymatic activity assay).
  - *GBA1* genotyping is difficult due to the proximity of the highly homologous pseudogene *GBAP1*, which shares over 96% of its exons with *GBA1*.
  - Mutation analysis in a limited panel with heterogeneous affected alleles may miss pathogenic variants or fail to rule out the disease.
  - DNA sequencing of the entire glucocerebrosidase (*GBA1*) coding region using next-generation sequencing (NGS), followed by confirmation through Sanger sequencing, is a reliable method for detecting point mutations in individuals suspected of Gaucher disease (GD) without known affected family members. Detection of recombinant alleles may occur between the gene and pseudogene [41].
  - Identification of deficient glucocerebrosidase enzyme activity is recommended for individuals with biallelic GBA1 pathogenic variants to confirm the diagnosis and verify the segregation of pathogenic variant alleles [6].
  - Multiplex ligation-probe amplification (MLPA) and messenger ribonucleic acid (mRNA) analysis should be conducted to identify potential unidentified recombinant or deleted alleles and deep intronic pathogenic variants under two conditions, respectively: the lack of homozygous

pathogenic variants in parents and the absence of pathogenic variants (in one or both alleles) after sequencing [42].
- Saposin C deficiency should be considered in the presence of the clinical phenotype and biochemical findings compatible with GD and normal or low BGLU activity in cells but without a pathologic variant in the *GBA* gene (Fig. 4.4).
- Dried blood spot (DBS) is a highly convenient and popular method for diagnosing Gaucher disease.
- Acid β-glucocerebrosidase activity and glucosylsphingosine levels can be assessed in DBS, but the positive predictive value is low and requires further research.
- The results should be interpreted carefully due to challenges in sample storage and delivery, as well as a lack of correlation between standard and DBS assays and specificity.
- Diagnosis of Gaucher disease via DBS (assessing enzyme activity or glucosylsphingosine levels) should be confirmed by identifying biallelic pathogenic variants in the *GBA1* gene (Fig. 4.4) [6].

- **Prediction and Classification of Clinical Course.**
  Genetic studies can help classify patients and predict clinical outcomes, but genotype-phenotype correlations in GD are often imperfect. The significant overlap in clinical manifestations among patients with different genotypes complicates genetic counseling, although some genotype-phenotype correlations have been identified (Table 4.1) [43]:
  - Patients with GD1 who carry at least one p.Asn409Ser allele do not exhibit neurological symptoms, but the risk of Parkinson's disease must still be considered [44].
  - The homozygous variant for the p.Asn409Ser or p.Arg535His is related to milder GD type 1, while some individuals experience progressive disease. Some Ashkenazi Jewish patients with this variant may be asymptomatic [45].
  - The homozygous variant p.Leu483Pro is linked to an unstable enzyme that has minimal or no residual activity. In patients with GD2 and GD3, this variant is associated with neurologic complications, although some adult patients with this genotype have not experienced any significant neurologic issues [44].
  - In patients with myoclonic epilepsy associated with GD, the variants p.Val433Leu (V394L), p.Gly416Ser (G377S), and p.Asn227Ser (N188S) have been identified, alongside p.Leu483Pro and other alleles related to neuropathic GD [46].
  - Homozygous for the p.Asp448His variant (commonly known as the D409H allele) is associated with cardiovascular and corneal involvement in GD3c [47].
  - The mutated alleles p.Ser235Pro (S196P), p.Arg170Leu (R131L), p.Arg159Trp (R120W), and p.Arg296Gln (R257Q), along with compound heterozygosity for a pathogenic insertion type, were reported in collodion babies [48].
  - The pathogenic missense variant p.Arg159Gln (R120Q) is linked to the perinatal-lethal form GD [49].
  - Patients with compound heterozygotes c.[84dupG] + [115 + 1G > A] experience subacute disease progression resulting in progressive pulmonary disease, often leading to death in the first or second decade. In contrast, the homozygous variant is lethal [22].
  - The c.1226A > G (N370S) mutation is common in the Ashkenazi Jewish population, found in 75–80% of GD1 alleles. Both homozygous and heterozygous variants eliminate the risk of neurological disorders (GD2, GD3), although they do not predict the severity of bone and visceral involvement. Approximately 75% of GD1 patients who develop symptoms after age 50 have the N370S/N370S genotype [50],

Table 4.1 Some proposed phenotype-genotype correlation in GD

Variant	Erlenmeyer flask	Bone pain	Osteopenia	Anemia, thrombocy topenia	Hepatomegaly	Splenomegaly	Myoclonic seizure	Prenatal fatal	Corneal involvement	Clodion baby	Cardiac involvement	No symptom	GD3	GD2	GD1
p.Asn409Ser (c.1226A > G) (N370S)	–	–	–	–	–	–	–	–	–	–	–	–	–	–	+
p. Arg535His (c.1604G > A)	–	–	–	–	–	–	–	–	–	–	–	–	–	–	+
p. Leu483Pro (c.1448 T > C) (L44P)	–	–	–	–	–	–	–	–	–	–	–	–	+	+	–
p.Asp448His (D409H)	–	–	–	–	–	–	–	–	+	–	+	–	+	–	–
p. Val433Leu (V394L)	–	–	–	–	–	–	+	–	–	–	–	–	–	–	–
p. Gly416Ser (G377S)	–	–	–	–	–	–	+	–	–	–	–	–	–	–	–
p. Asn227Ser (N188S)	–	–	–	–	–	–	+	–		–	–	–	–	–	–
p.Arg170Leu (R131L)	–	–	–	-	–	–	–	–	–	+	–	–	–	–	–
p. Ser235Pro (S196P)	–	–	–	–	–	–	–	–	–	+	–	–	–	–	–
p.Arg159Trp (R120W)	–	–	–	–	–	–	–	–	–	+	–	–	–	–	–
p.Arg296Gln (R257Q9)	–	–	–	–	–	–	–	–	–	+	–	–	–	–	–
p. Arg159Gln (R120Q)	–	–	–	–		–	–	+	–	–	–	–	–	–	–
N370S/84GG	+	+	–	+	+	+	–	–	–	–	–	–	–	–	+
N370S/N370S	–	–	–	–	+	+	–	–	–	–	–	+	–	–	+
N370S/L444P	+	+	–	–	+	+	–	–	–	–	–	–	–	–	–
N370S/others	+	–	+	–	–	–	–	–	–	–	–	–	–	–	–

with half of these individuals likely never seeking medical care. For children under 18 with this genotype, the median age of onset is 10 years [51].

- A deletion of 55 base pairs (Δ55) in exon 9 may be misinterpreted as N370S homozygosity rather than N370S/Δ55. Patients with this deletion display the same phenotype as those with N370S/84GG or N370S/null [52].
- The homozygous L444P variant significantly increases the risk of neurological impairment (GD2, 3) [53]. Patients with two null mutations, leading to a complete lack of glucocerebrosidase activity, do not survive beyond the perinatal period due to fetal forms incompatible with life.
- Massive hepatomegaly (≥2.5 MN) is rare in patients with N370S/L444P, N370S/N370S, and N370S/other genotypes. In contrast, those with N370S/84GG and other genotypes exhibit similar hepatomegaly characteristics, with approximately 30% having livers ≥2.5 MN [54].
- Some patients with the N370S/N370S variant have massive spleens (≥15 MN), and many patients with spleens ≤5 MN (28%) are affected by the genotype N370S/N370S. Spleens in N370S/84GG patients are significantly larger, with nearly 70% having volume ≥ 15 MN and none below ≤5 MN.
- Moderate thrombocytopenia and anemia are the most common hematologic findings even in the presence of massive splenic enlargement in N370S/84GG patients.
- The largest percentage (~30%) of patients with osteopenia had the genotypes Unknown or N370S/Other, and osteopenia was low (~17%) in N370S homozygotes.
- Erlenmeyer flask deformities occurred in about 78% of N370S/84GG patients, while the N370S/L444P and N370S/Other groups had about 43% Erlenmeyer flask deformities. The greatest proportions of bone pain were reported in the N370S/84GG and N370S/L444P genotypes [54].

- **Carrier Detection.**
  Mutation analysis using Sanger sequencing can identify the siblings and parents of affected patients.
- **Prenatal Diagnosis.**
  Two methods for prenatal diagnosis have been recommended:
  - Enzyme analysis conducted using fetal cells from chorionic villus sampling or amniocentesis [55].
  - Genetic analysis through chorionic villus sampling (sampled at 10–12 weeks of gestational age) or amniotic fluid cells (as early as 16 weeks of gestational age). Awareness of DNA mutations in the proband or heterozygous parents enables the use of DNA mutation and enzyme analysis for prenatal identification [56].

Newborn Screening (NBS)

NBS for detection lysosomal storage disease has been performed by measuring beta-glucosidase activity on dried blood spots through tandem mass spectrometry, fluorometric, and digital microfluidics methods in some countries [57–61]. NBS prevents delayed diagnosis and initiates treatment.

The effectiveness of NBS in detecting GD is debated due to incomplete correlations between genotype and phenotype, highlighting the need for the further understanding of individual genetic codes. Targeted NBS based on family history and ethnicity may be practical for early detection and ERT [62].

Learning Points

- Diagnosis of GD methods include enzyme assays, biochemical tests, bone marrow aspiration, and molecular studies.
- Genetic analysis is used for the confirmation of diagnosis, the prediction and classification of the clinical course, carrier detection, and prenatal diagnosis.

References

1. Beutler E, Saven A. Misuse of marrow examination in the diagnosis of Gaucher disease. Blood. 1990;76(3):646–8.
2. Verma J, Thomas DC, Sharma S, Jhingan G, Singh A, Hsiao KJ, et al. Inherited metabolic disorders: quality management for laboratory diagnosis. Clin Chim Acta. 2015;447:1–7.
3. Choy FY, Davidson RG. Gaucher's disease II. Studies on the kinetics of beta-glucosidase and the effects of sodium taurocholate in normal and Gaucher tissues. Pediatr Res. 1980;14(1):54–9.
4. Herrera D, Monaga M, Campos D, Pampín Y, González EC, Lavaut K. Ultramicro-fluorometric assay for the diagnosis of Gaucher disease in dried blood spots on filter paper. J Neonatal Perinatal Med. 2013;6(1):61–7.
5. Turner BM, Hirschhorn K. Properties of beta-glucosidase in cultured skin fibroblasts from controls and patients with Gaucher disease. Am J Hum Genet. 1978;30(4):346–58.
6. Dardis A, Michelakakis H, Rozenfeld P, Fumic K, Wagner J, Pavan E, et al. Patient centered guidelines for the laboratory diagnosis of Gaucher disease type 1. Orphanet J Rare Dis. 2022;17(1):442.
7. Schmitz M, Alfalah M, Aerts JM, Naim HY, Zimmer KP. Impaired trafficking of mutants of lysosomal glucocerebrosidase in Gaucher's disease. Int J Biochem Cell Biol. 2005;37(11):2310–20.
8. Wenger DA, Clark C, Sattler M, Wharton C. Synthetic substrate beta-glucosidase activity in leukocytes: a reproducible method for the identification of patients and carriers of Gaucher's disease. Clin Genet. 1978;13(2):145–53.
9. Berger J, Lecourt S, Vanneaux V, Rapatel C, Boisgard S, Caillaud C, et al. Glucocerebrosidase deficiency dramatically impairs human bone marrow haematopoiesis in an in vitro model of Gaucher disease. Br J Haematol. 2010;150(1):93–101.
10. Charrow J, Andersson HC, Kaplan P, Kolodny EH, Mistry P, Pastores G, et al. The Gaucher registry: demographics and disease characteristics of 1698 patients with Gaucher disease. Arch Intern Med. 2000;160(18):2835–43.
11. Danilov SM, Tikhomirova VE, Metzger R, Naperova IA, Bukina TM, Goker-Alpan O, et al. ACE phenotyping in Gaucher disease. Mol Genet Metab. 2018;123(4):501–10.
12. Mekinian A, Stirnemann J, Belmatoug N, Heraoui D, Fantin B, Fain O, et al. Ferritinemia during type 1 Gaucher disease: mechanisms and progression under treatment. Blood Cells Mol Dis. 2012;49(1):53–7.
13. Stein P, Yu H, Jain D, Mistry PK. Hyperferritinemia and iron overload in type 1 Gaucher disease. Am J Hematol. 2010;85(7):472–6.
14. Kadir RA, Kingman CE, Chi C, O'Connell NM, Riddell A, Lee CA, et al. Screening for factor XI deficiency amongst pregnant women of Ashkenazi Jewish origin. Haemophilia. 2006;12(6):625–8.
15. Wine E, Yaniv I, Cohen IJ. Hyperimmunoglobulinemia in pediatric-onset type 1 Gaucher disease and effects of enzyme replacement therapy. J Pediatr Hematol Oncol. 2007;29(7):451–7.
16. van Dussen L, Hendriks EJ, Groener JE, Boot RG, Hollak CE, Aerts JM. Value of plasma chitotriosidase to assess non-neuronopathic Gaucher disease severity and progression in the era of enzyme replacement therapy. J Inherit Metab Dis. 2014;37(6):991–1001.
17. Hollak CE, van Weely S, van Oers MH, Aerts JM. Marked elevation of plasma chitotriosidase activity. A novel hallmark of Gaucher disease. J Clin Invest. 1994;93(3):1288–92.
18. Boot RG, Renkema GH, Verhoek M, Strijland A, Bliek J, de Meulemeester TM, et al. The human chitotriosidase gene. Nature of inherited enzyme deficiency. J Biol Chem. 1998;273(40):25680–5.
19. Bargagli E, Bennett D, Maggiorelli C, Di Sipio P, Margollicci M, Bianchi N, et al. Human chitotriosidase: a sensitive biomarker of sarcoidosis. J Clin Immunol. 2013;33(1):264–70.
20. Bellinghausen I, Reuter S, Martin H, Maxeiner J, Luxemburger U, Türeci Ö, et al. Enhanced production of CCL18 by tolerogenic dendritic cells is associated with inhibition of allergic airway reactivity. J Allergy Clin Immunol. 2012;130(6):1384–93.
21. Boot RG, Verhoek M, de Fost M, Hollak CE, Maas M, Bleijlevens B, et al. Marked elevation of the chemokine CCL18/PARC in Gaucher disease: a novel surrogate marker for assessing therapeutic intervention. Blood. 2004;103(1):33–9.
22. Stirnemann J, Belmatoug N, Camou F, Serratrice C, Froissart R, Caillaud C, et al. A review of Gaucher disease pathophysiology, clinical presentation and treatments. Int J Mol Sci. 2017;18(2)
23. Deegan PB, Moran MT, McFarlane I, Schofield JP, Boot RG, Aerts JM, et al. Clinical evaluation of chemokine and enzymatic biomarkers of Gaucher disease. Blood Cells Mol Dis. 2005;35(2):259–67.
24. Dimitriou E, Verhoek M, Altun S, Karabatsos F, Moraitou M, Youssef J, et al. Elevated plasma chemokine CCL18/PARC in beta-thalassemia. Blood Cells Mol Dis. 2005;35(3):328–31.
25. Irún P, Cebolla JJ, López de Frutos L, De Castro-Orós I, Roca-Espiau M, Giraldo P. LC-MS/MS analysis of plasma glucosylsphingosine as a biomarker for diagnosis and follow-up monitoring in Gaucher disease in the Spanish population. Clin Chem Lab Med. 2020;58(5):798–809.
26. Rolfs A, Giese AK, Grittner U, Mascher D, Elstein D, Zimran A, et al. Glucosylsphingosine is a highly sensitive and specific biomarker for primary diagnostic and follow-up monitoring in Gaucher disease in a non-Jewish, Caucasian cohort of Gaucher disease patients. PLoS One. 2013;8(11):e79732.

27. Dekker N, van Dussen L, Hollak CE, Overkleeft H, Scheij S, Ghauharali K, et al. Elevated plasma glucosylsphingosine in Gaucher disease: relation to phenotype, storage cell markers, and therapeutic response. Blood. 2011;118(16):e118–27.
28. Ferraz MJ, Marques AR, Gaspar P, Mirzaian M, van Roomen C, Ottenhoff R, et al. Lyso-glycosphingolipid abnormalities in different murine models of lysosomal storage disorders. Mol Genet Metab. 2016;117(2):186–93.
29. Gaspar P, Kallemeijn WW, Strijland A, Scheij S, Van Eijk M, Aten J, et al. Action myoclonus-renal failure syndrome: diagnostic applications of activity-based probes and lipid analysis. J Lipid Res. 2014;55(1):138–45.
30. Motta M, Tatti M, Furlan F, Celato A, Di Fruscio G, Polo G, et al. Clinical, biochemical and molecular characterization of prosaposin deficiency. Clin Genet. 2016;90(3):220–9.
31. Murugesan V, Chuang WL, Liu J, Lischuk A, Kacena K, Lin H, et al. Glucosylsphingosine is a key biomarker of Gaucher disease. Am J Hematol. 2016;91(11):1082–9.
32. van Breemen MJ, de Fost M, Voerman JS, Laman JD, Boot RG, Maas M, et al. Increased plasma macrophage inflammatory protein (MIP)-1alpha and MIP-1beta levels in type 1 Gaucher disease. Biochim Biophys Acta. 2007;1772(7):788–96.
33. Aerts JM, Kallemeijn WW, Wegdam W, Joao Ferraz M, van Breemen MJ, Dekker N, et al. Biomarkers in the diagnosis of lysosomal storage disorders: proteins, lipids, and inhibodies. J Inherit Metab Dis. 2011;34(3):605–19.
34. Ivanova M, Dao J, Noll L, Fikry J, Goker-Alpan O. TRAP5b and RANKL/OPG predict bone pathology in patients with Gaucher disease. J Clin Med. 2021;10(10)
35. van der Lienden MJC, Gaspar P, Boot R, Aerts J, van Eijk M, Glycoprotein Non-Metastatic Protein B. An emerging biomarker for lysosomal dysfunction in macrophages. Int J Mol Sci. 2018;20(1)
36. Marcucci G, Zimran A, Bembi B, Kanis J, Reginster JY, Rizzoli R, et al. Gaucher disease and bone manifestations. Calcif Tissue Int. 2014;95(6):477–94.
37. de Fost M, Langeveld M, Franssen R, Hutten BA, Groener JE, de Groot E, et al. Low HDL cholesterol levels in type I Gaucher disease do not lead to an increased risk of cardiovascular disease. Atherosclerosis. 2009;204(1):267–72.
38. de Fost M, Out TA, de Wilde FA, Tjin EP, Pals ST, van Oers MH, et al. Immunoglobulin and free light chain abnormalities in Gaucher disease type I: data from an adult cohort of 63 patients and review of the literature. Ann Hematol. 2008;87(6):439–49.
39. Brautbar A, Elstein D, Pines G, Abrahamov A, Zimran A. Effect of enzyme replacement therapy on gammopathies in Gaucher disease. Blood Cells Mol Dis. 2004;32(1):214–7.
40. Yang HS, Cho KS, Park TS. Chronic myeloid leukemia with marked splenomegaly and pseudo-Gaucher cells. Blood Res. 2013;48(4):241.
41. Hassan S, Lopez G, Stubblefield BK, Tayebi N, Sidransky E. Alleles with more than one mutation can complicate genotype/phenotype studies in Mendelian disorders: lessons from Gaucher disease. Mol Genet Metab. 2018;125(1–2):1–3.
42. Amico G, Grossi S, Vijzelaar R, Lanza F, Mazzotti R, Corsolini F, et al. MLPA-based approach for initial and simultaneous detection of GBA deletions and recombinant alleles in patients affected by Gaucher disease. Mol Genet Metab. 2016;119(4):329–37.
43. Biegstraaten M, van Schaik IN, Aerts JM, Langeveld M, Mannens MM, Bour LJ, et al. A monozygotic twin pair with highly discordant Gaucher phenotypes. Blood Cells Mol Dis. 2011;46(1):39–41.
44. Koprivica V, Stone DL, Park JK, Callahan M, Frisch A, Cohen IJ, et al. Analysis and classification of 304 mutant alleles in patients with type 1 and type 3 Gaucher disease. Am J Hum Genet. 2000;66(6):1777–86.
45. Bronstein S, Karpati M, Peleg L. An update of Gaucher mutations distribution in the Ashkenazi Jewish population: prevalence and country of origin of the mutation R496H. Isr Med Assoc J. 2014;16(11):683–5.
46. Park JK, Orvisky E, Tayebi N, Kaneski C, Lamarca ME, Stubblefield BK, et al. Myoclonic epilepsy in Gaucher disease: genotype-phenotype insights from a rare patient subgroup. Pediatr Res. 2003;53(3):387–95.
47. Michelakakis H, Skardoutsou A, Mathioudakis J, Moraitou M, Dimitriou E, Voudris C, et al. Early-onset severe neurological involvement and D409H homozygosity in Gaucher disease: outcome of enzyme replacement therapy. Blood Cells Mol Dis. 2002;28(1):1–4.
48. Stone DL, Carey WF, Christodoulou J, Sillence D, Nelson P, Callahan M, et al. Type 2 Gaucher disease: the collodion baby phenotype revisited. Arch Dis Child Fetal Neonatal Ed. 2000;82(2):F163–6.
49. Felderhoff-Mueser U, Uhl J, Penzel R, Van Landeghem F, Vogel M, Obladen M, et al. Intrauterine onset of acute neuropathic type 2 Gaucher disease: identification of a novel insertion sequence. Am J Med Genet A. 2004;128a(2):138–43.
50. Balwani M, Fuerstman L, Kornreich R, Edelmann L, Desnick RJ. Type 1 Gaucher disease: significant disease manifestations in "asymptomatic" homozygotes. Arch Intern Med. 2010;170(16):1463–9.
51. Kaplan P, Andersson HC, Kacena KA, Yee JD. The clinical and demographic characteristics of nonneuronopathic Gaucher disease in 887 children at diagnosis. Arch Pediatr Adolesc Med. 2006;160(6):603–8.
52. Walley AJ, Harris A. A novel point mutation (D380A) and a rare deletion (1255del55) in the glucocerebrosidase gene causing Gaucher's disease. Hum Mol Genet. 1993;2(10):1737–8.

53. Cindik N, Ozcay F, Süren D, Akkoyun I, Gökdemir M, Varan B, et al. Gaucher disease with communicating hydrocephalus and cardiac involvement. Clin Cardiol. 2010;33(1):E26–30.
54. Grabowski GA, Zimran A, Ida H. Gaucher disease types 1 and 3: phenotypic characterization of large populations from the ICGG Gaucher registry. Am J Hematol. 2015;90(Suppl 1):S12–8.
55. Singh Y, Arora D, Kochar S. Prenatal diagnosis of Gaucher disease. Med J Armed Forces India. 2010;66(2):170–1.
56. Yoshida S, Kido J, Matsumoto S, Momosaki K, Mitsubuchi H, Shimazu T, et al. Prenatal diagnosis of Gaucher disease using next-generation sequencing. Pediatr Int. 2016;58(9):946–9.
57. Han M, Jun SH, Song SH, Park KU, Kim JQ, Song J. Use of tandem mass spectrometry for newborn screening of 6 lysosomal storage disorders in a Korean population. Korean J Lab Med. 2011;31(4):250–6.
58. Kang L, Zhan X, Gu X, Zhang H. Successful newborn screening for Gaucher disease using fluorometric assay in China. J Hum Genet. 2017;62(8):763–8.
59. Liao HC, Chiang CC, Niu DM, Wang CH, Kao SM, Tsai FJ, et al. Detecting multiple lysosomal storage diseases by tandem mass spectrometry–a national newborn screening program in Taiwan. Clin Chim Acta 2014;431:80–86.
60. Sista RS, Wang T, Wu N, Graham C, Eckhardt A, Bali D, et al. Rapid assays for Gaucher and hurler diseases in dried blood spots using digital microfluidics. Mol Genet Metab. 2013;109(2):218–20.
61. Wittmann J, Karg E, Turi S, Legnini E, Wittmann G, Giese AK, et al. Newborn screening for lysosomal storage disorders in Hungary. JIMD Rep. 2012;6:117–25.
62. Zimran A, Altarescu G, Elstein D. Screening for Gaucher disease: new challenges. Isr Med Assoc J. 2014;16(11):723–4.
63. Mistry PK, Cappellini MD, Lukina E, Özsan H, Pascual SM, et al. A reappraisal of Gaucher disease – diagnosis and disease management algorithms. AJH. 2011;86(1):110–5.

5 Overview Assessment of Gaucher Disease

Maryam Asgharnejad and Parastoo Rostami

5.1 Initial Assessment of Gaucher Disease

Baseline (pretreatment) assessments are essential for patients with GD due to the variability in disease manifestations, severity, and progression. Additionally, this evaluation aids in treatment plan selection. Recommended parameters for this assessment include the following (Fig. 5.1).

5.1.1 Family and Medical History

- Family history of ethnicity and consanguinity, along with history of GD in parents and/or siblings.
- History of Parkinson's disease or Lewy body dementia in parents, grandparents, or siblings.
- History of splenectomy, blood transfusions, bone pain, pathologic fractures, dyspnea, bleeding tendency, and/or perinatal deaths/hydrops fetalis [1, 2].

5.1.2 Clinical and Paraclinical Examination

- Physical and clinical examination, including palpation of the abdomen for liver and spleen enlargement, offer valuable insights for physicians to evaluate disease severity and extent.

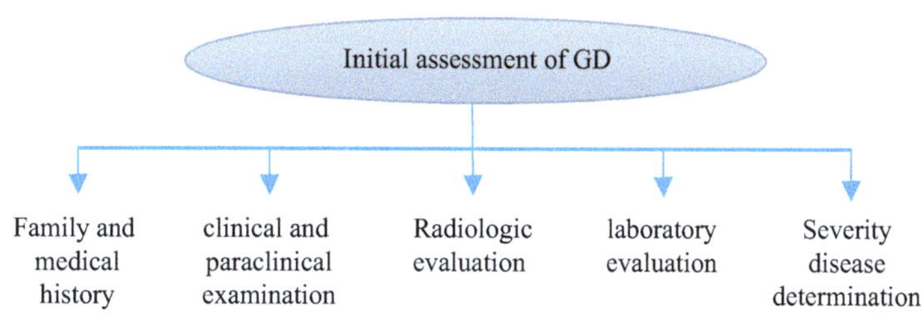

Fig. 5.1 Initial assessment of GD

M. Asgharnejad
Farateb Ayeen Institute, Tehran, Iran

P. Rostami (✉)
Research Center for Growth and Development, Division of Endocrinology and Metabolism, Department of Pediatrics, Pediatrics Center of Excellence, Tehran University of Medical Sciences, Tehran, Iran

© The Author(s), under exclusive license to Springer Nature Singapore Pte Ltd. 2025
P. Rostami, A. Talea (eds.), *Gaucher Disease*, https://doi.org/10.1007/978-981-96-4763-7_5

- Assessing weight, height, and head circumference against age and sex-standardized growth charts can determine the presence of growth retardation.
- An ophthalmologist must examine the eyes for strabismus and abnormal extraocular movements.
- Assessing the development of puberty in adolescence to determine the severity and duration of the disease is useful [1–3].
- Cardiopulmonary involvement is one of the rare but serious complications in children with GD and should be included in the baseline evaluation program.
  Children with compound heterozygotes variants and patients carrying the c.84insG or IVS2 + 1 variant are more likely to have progressive pulmonary involvement.
  Pulmonary hypertension occurs in adults with GD1, and risk factors for severe pulmonary hypertension include family history of pulmonary hypertension, asplenia, female sex, and angiotensin-converting enzyme (ACE) I gene polymorphism. The D409H/D409H variant is related to cardiac valvular involvement in GD3.
  Cardiopulmonary function is evaluated by chest radiograph, high-resolution computed tomography thoracic imaging, echocardiogram electrocardiogram, and pulmonary function tests (forced vital capacity and forced expiratory volume in one second (FEV1)) [4].
- Neurologic involvement is an important complication in patients with GD1, especially GD2 and GD3.
  Evaluation of the neurologic system is essential to determine the prognosis and treatment after diagnosis.
  An experienced neurologist in GD should examine patients for neurological involvement. Brain imaging, preferably magnetic resonance imaging (MRI) or computed tomography (CT), may be needed in some situations [5].
- Assessment of peripheral hearing has been recommended by different methods, including electroacoustic emission in small children and pure tone audiometry in older patients [6]. Abnormalities of brainstem-evoked potential in GD3 correlate with cognitive dysfunction and disease severity [7].

5.1.3 Radiological Evaluation

Radiologic surveys can aid in treatment planning, disease prognosis, and therapy response monitoring. Initial radiologic studies include the following:

- MRI: MRI (coronal T1- and T2-weighted scans) of the lumbar spine and femoral head is used to identify bone involvement, including marrow infiltration, bone crises, osteonecrosis, and infarction. T1-weighted MRI is particularly effective for detecting bone marrow infiltration, while T2-weighted MRI is the most sensitive for active bone infarcts [1, 2, 4].
- Radiographs: compression fractures of the spine and femoral head, as well as other skeletal disease, can sometimes be asymptomatic. Therefore, plain radiographs—specifically the anteroposterior view of the femora and lateral view of the spine—are useful for detecting skeletal involvement. Additionally, radiographs of other bone sites may be performed based on symptoms.
  Bone age X-rays can be helpful in assessing puberty during adolescence [8, 9]. In children suspected of having GD3, chest X-rays can reveal lung involvement.
- DXA: dual-energy X-ray absorptiometry (DXA) of the lumbar spine and femoral neck assesses osteopenia severity but requires careful interpretation [10].

5.1.4 Laboratory Evaluation

- Measure white blood cell (WBC) count, hemoglobin concentration, platelet count, electrolytes, and serum iron and ferritin. Also, perform liver function tests, thyroid function tests, and coagulation studies.

- Serum electrophoresis and free light chains should also be assessed at baseline to evaluate adults clonal gammopathies. Biomarkers such as chitotriosidase or C-C motif chemokine ligand 18 (CCL18)/pulmonary and activation-regulated chemokine (PARC) and glucosylsphingosine should be measured at baseline and periodically during treatment.
- Other biochemical studies involve measuring serum calcium, phosphorous, alkaline phosphatase, concentrations of vitamin D and parathyroid hormone, and alpha-fetoprotein (AFP).

5.1.5 Determining Disease Severity

Determining the severity of the disease is useful for assessing its activity, determining and adjusting the dose of enzyme replacement therapy (ERT), and monitoring treatment. The first severity score index for Gaucher type 1 (Zimran SSI) was introduced by Zimran et al. in 1992 [11].

Subsequently, in 2008, Maja Di Rocco et al. released a new Gaucher severity score index for assessing disease activity, staging, and treatment response (GauSSI-I).

GauSSI-I consists of 42 points across six different domains, each with varied weighted parameters [12] (Table. 5.1):

- Skeletal domain (bone marrow infiltration and bone mineral component subdomains) (maximum combined score: 11).
- Hematologic domain (maximum score: 10).
- Biomarker domain (maximum score: 3).
- Visceral domain (maximum score: 11).
- Lung domain (maximum score: 4).
- Neurological domain (maximum score: 3).

Bone marrow infiltration assessment is not validated in children, allowing for the use of GauSSI-I in adult patients.

Bone Marrow Infiltration Subdomain

Bone marrow infiltration scores for the bone marrow component are assessed by MRI and scintigraphy. The data should be interpreted by an expert radiologist in GD (Table 5.2) [12].

Bone Mineral Subdomain

Bone mineral assessment is a key component of the skeletal domain used for the scoring severity system. Bone mineral involvement has been categorized into four groups: lack of lesions (score 0), mild involvement (grade 1), intermediate severity (grade 2), and severe involvement (grade 3).

Bone mineral assessment through DEXA, as T-score (relationship with healthy individuals at the peak of BMD) −1 and − 2.5 and with Z-score (relationship with healthy individuals of the same age) −1.5 threshold level has been considered (Table 5.3) [12].

Bone mineral assessment is a key component of the skeletal scoring system, categorized into four groups: no lesions (score 0), mild involvement (grade 1), intermediate involvement (grade 2), and severe involvement (grade 3).

Bone mineral density (BMD) is measured by DEXA, with T-scores comparing results to the peak BMD of healthy adults and Z-scores comparing results to age-matched individuals.

Learning Points

- An initial assessment of Gaucher disease is essential for developing a treatment plan.
- This assessment includes evaluations of family and medical history, clinical and paraclinical examinations, radiological and laboratory evaluations, and determination of disease severity.

Table 5.1 Gaucher severity score index for the evaluation of disease activity, staging, and response to treatment (GauSSI-I)

Skeletal domain		Hematologic domain		Visceral domain	
Bone marrow infiltration (based on either MRI or scintigraphy evaluation)		**Hemoglobin concentration**		**[a]Spleen**	
Absent/minimal	0	>12 g/dl (male), >11.5 (female)	0	No MRI/US lesion	0
Mild	1	Between 10 and 12 g/dl	1	MR/US lesion	3
Intermediate	2	Between 8 and 9.9 g/dl	2	No splenectomy	0
Severe	3	<8 g/dl	3	Splenectomy	2
		Or < 8g/dl or need for blood transfusion		Volume < 5 N	0
Impairment of mineral component (based on either DEXA or Hemann's X-ray)		**White blood cell count**		Between 5 and 9 N	1
Absent/minimal	0	$>4 \times 10^9$/L	0	Between 10 and 15 N	2
Mild	1	Between 2.5×10^9/L	1 a/b	Volume > 15 N	3
Intermediate	2	$<2.5 \times 10^9$/L	2 a/b		
Severe	3	$<1.9 \times 10^9$/L	3 a/b		
Osteonecrosis		**Platelet count**		**[b]Liver**	
None	0	>150 × 109/L	0	No hepatic disease	0
Medullary infarction	1	Between 101 and 150 × 109/L	1 a/b	Hepatic disease 3	3
Osteonecrosis	2	Between 60 and 100 × 109/L	2 a/b	Volume < 1.25 N	0
Prosthesis	3	<60 × 109/L	3 a/b	Between 1.25–25 N	1
Pathologic fractures		**Bleeding time**		Volume > 2.5 N	2
Absent	0	< 8 min	0		
Reported	2	> 8 min	1		

Lung domain		Biomarker domain		Neurological domain	
Pulmonary hypertension		**[d]Serum chitotriosidase or CCL18**			
Absent	0	Chitotriosidase <600 nmol/ml × h	Score 0	No signs/symptoms	0
Moderate	1	Chitotriosidase 600–4000 nmol/ml × h	Score 1	Peripheral neuropathy	1
Severe	2	Chitotriosidase 4001–15,000 nmol/ml × h	Score 2	Parkinson's disease/ parkinsonism	3
[c]Respiratory failure		Chitotriosidase >15,000 nmol/ml × h	Score 3		
Absent	0	CCL18 < 72 ng/ml	Score 0		

(continued)

Table 5.1 (continued)

Lung domain		Biomarker domain		Neurological domain	
Moderate	1	CCL18 < 72–236 ng/ml	Score 1		
Severe	2	CCL18 237–1000 ng/ml	Score 2		
		CCL18 > 1000 ng/ml	Score 3		

a: nonsplenectomized patients, b: prior splenectomy, *NL* normal, *US* ultrasonography, *MR* magnetic resonance
[a]Splenomegaly is defined as a splenic mass greater than the normal 0.2% of total body weight in kilograms
[b]Hepatomegaly is defined as a liver mass greater than 1.25 times the normal 2.5% of total body weight in kilograms, and hepatomegaly >2.5 times normal is a severe risk factor for an untoward outcome of Gaucher disease
[c]Respiratory failure is employed after excluding possible concomitant causes of respiratory failure other than Gaucher disease documented by pulmonary function test
[d]The normal serum activity of chitotriosidase is 4–76 nmol/mL/hour, but in Gaucher disease, chitotriosidase levels increase to 300–65,000 nmol/mL/hour. The normal serum levels of CCL18 are between 10 and 72 ng/mL, and in the Gaucher population, a range of 237–2285 ng/mL (with a median of 948 ng/mL) has been reported. Only one biomarker (either chitotriosidase or CCL18/PARC) is employed in GauSSI-I, and chitotriosidase is used only after the exclusion of homozygous or heterozygous mutations (174)

Table 5.2 New categories of disease severity (normalized score, first column on the left of each panel) proposed for magnetic resonance evaluation and for scintigraphy evaluation of bone marrow involvement in patients with Gaucher disease [12]

Normalized	Rosenthal score	Dusseldorf score	Terk score	VDR score	BMB score
0	0	0	0	>2	0–2
1	1–3	1–3	1a/b	1.5–2	3–7
2	4–7	4–6	2a/b	1–1.5	8–12
3	8–11	7–8	3a/b	<1	13–16
Normalized score	QCSI fat fraction	S-MRI score	99mTc-sestamibi	99mTc-radiocolloid score	
0	>3	0–4	0–2	Normal	
1	0.30–0.25	5–10	3–4	Mild	
2	0.20–0.25	11–17	5–6	Moderate	
3	<0.20	18–24	7–8	Severe	

S-MRI Spanish magnetic resonance index, *VDR* vertebral disk ratio, *BMB* bone marrow burden, *QCSI* quantitative chemical shift index

Table 5.3 Bone mineral subdomain new categories of disease severity [12]

Normalized	Hermann's X-ray score	Z-score	DEXA BMD T-score
0	0	1 < Z < 0	T > 0
1	1	1–3	0 < T < −1
2	2–3	4–6	−1 < T < −2.5
3	4–5	7–8	T < - 2.5
Additional score	Osteonecrosis	Pathological fractures	
0	None	Absent	
1	Medullary infarction		
2	Osteonecrosis	Present	
3	Prosthesis		

References

1. Charrow J, Andersson HC, Kaplan P, Kolodny EH, Mistry P, Pastores G, et al. Enzyme replacement therapy and monitoring for children with type 1 Gaucher disease: consensus recommendations. J Pediatr. 2004;144(1):112–20.
2. Grabowski GA, Andria G, Baldellou A, Campbell PE, Charrow J, Cohen IJ, et al. Pediatric non-neuronopathic Gaucher disease: presentation, diagnosis and assessment. Consensus statements. Eur J Pediatr. 2004;163(2):58–66.
3. Tayebi N, Walker J, Stubblefield B, Orvisky E, LaMarca ME, Wong K, et al. Gaucher disease with parkinsonian manifestations: does glucocerebrosidase deficiency contribute to a vulnerability to parkinsonism? Mol Genet Metab. 2003;79(2):104–9.
4. Weinreb NJ, Aggio MC, Andersson HC, Andria G, Charrow J, Clarke JT, et al. Gaucher disease type 1: revised recommendations on evaluations and monitoring for adult patients. Semin Hematol. 2004;41(4 Suppl 5):15–22.
5. Vellodi A, Bembi B, de Villemeur TB, Collin-Histed T, Erikson A, Mengel E, et al. Management of neuronopathic Gaucher disease: a European consensus. J Inherit Metab Dis. 2001;24(3):319–27.
6. Bamiou DE, Campbell P, Liasis A, Page J, Sirimanna T, Boyd S, et al. Audiometric abnormalities in children with Gaucher disease type 3. Neuropediatrics. 2001;32(3):136–41.
7. Tantawy AA, Sherif EM, Adly AA, Hassanine S, Awad AH. Evoked potentials and neurocognitive functions in pediatric Egyptian Gaucher patients on enzyme replacement therapy: a single center experience. J Inherit Metab Dis. 2013;36(6):1025–37.
8. Maas M, Poll LW, Terk MR. Imaging and quantifying skeletal involvement in Gaucher disease. Br J Radiol. 2002;75(Suppl 1):A13–24.
9. Ross DJ, Spira S, Buchbinder NA. Gaucher cells in pulmonary-capillary blood in association with pulmonary hypertension. N Engl J Med. 1997;336(5):379–81.
10. Crabtree NJ, Kibirige MS, Fordham JN, Banks LM, Muntoni F, Chinn D, et al. The relationship between lean body mass and bone mineral content in paediatric health and disease. Bone. 2004;35(4):965–72.
11. Zimran A, Kay A, Gelbart T, Garver P, Thurston D, Saven A, et al. Gaucher disease. Clinical, laboratory, radiologic, and genetic features of 53 patients. Medicine (Baltimore). 1992;71(6):337–53.
12. Di Rocco M, Giona F, Carubbi F, Linari S, Minichilli F, Brady RO, et al. A new severity score index for phenotypic classification and evaluation of responses to treatment in type I Gaucher disease. Haematologica. 2008;93(8):1211–8.

Overview Treatment of Gaucher Disease

6

Nima Parvaneh and Parastoo Rostami

6.1 Introduction

Gaucher disease (GD) was the first inherited metabolic disorder treated with enzyme replacement therapy (ERT). The management of GD should ideally involve a multidisciplinary team.

Before initiating treatment, it is essential to establish treatment goals, which generally include symptom improvement, the prevention of irreversible complications, and the enhancement of overall health and quality of life. In children, also consider maintaining or reversing optimal growth. Recommended management and treatment for all types of GD include the following:

- **Goal of Treatment for GD**
  - Management goals of long-term complications.
  - Short-term management goals.
  - Long-term management goals.
- **Choice of Treatment for GD**
  - Enzyme replacement therapy (ERT).
  - Substrate reduction therapy (SRT).
  - Splenectomy.
  - Hematopoietic stem cell transplantation (HSCT).
  - Gene therapy.
  - Enzymes enhancement therapy.
  - Noninhibitory chaperone agents.
  - Supportive care.

6.2 Goal of Treatment for GD

Therapeutic goals for optimal treatment established by international panels of experienced clinicians in GD include the following.

6.2.1 Management Goals of Long-Term Complications

- Early detection of hematologic malignancies such as multiple myeloma, lymphoma, and amyloidosis.
- Early detection of solid tumors (hepatocellular carcinoma and renal cell carcinoma).
- Early detection of parkinsonism/Parkinson's disease.
- Early detection of insulin resistance and type 2 diabetes mellitus [1].

N. Parvaneh
Division of Allergy and Clinical Immunology, Department of Pediatrics, Pediatrics Center of Excellence, Tehran University of Medical Sciences, Tehran, Iran
e-mail: nparvaneh@sina.tums.ac.ir

P. Rostami (✉)
Research Center for Growth and Development, Division of Endocrinology and Metabolism, Department of Pediatrics, Pediatrics Center of Excellence, Tehran University of Medical Sciences, Tehran, Iran

© The Author(s), under exclusive license to Springer Nature Singapore Pte Ltd. 2025
P. Rostami, A. Talea (eds.), *Gaucher Disease*, https://doi.org/10.1007/978-981-96-4763-7_6

6.2.2 Short-Term Management Goals

- Eliminate dependence on blood transfusions.
- Increase hemoglobin levels to over 11.0 g/dl for females and children and over 12.0 g/dl for males within 12–24 months.
- Increase platelet counts in the first year of treatment to prevent spontaneous bleeding.
- In patients who have undergone splenectomy, platelet counts normalize within 1 year of treatment.
- In patients with an intact spleen, achieve a platelet count of ≥100,000/mm^3 within 3 years of treatment.
- Reduce bone pain not associated with irreversible defects within 1–2 years.
- Decrease bone marrow involvement.
- Increase bone mineral density (BMD) by 2 years in adults with a baseline T-score below −2.5.
- Achieve normal skeletal mass in children.
- Achieve target height growth within 2 years of treatment.
- Avoid splenectomy.
- Reduce spleen volume to less than 2–8 times the baseline by years 1–2.
- Improve symptoms related to splenomegaly (e.g., abdominal distension, new splenic infarction).
- Reduce liver volume to 1–1.5 times the baseline within 1–2 years.
- Eliminate hypersplenism.
- Enhance quality-of-life scores from baseline within 2–3 years.
- Reduce fatigue not related to anemia.
- Improve physical function [1, 2].

6.2.3 Long-Term Management Goals for Gaucher Disease Type

- Maintain spleen volume less than two to eight times normal after years 1–2.
- Maintain normal or near normal liver volume after years 1–2.
- Prevent liver complications like fibrosis, cirrhosis, and portal hypertension.
- Maintain improved hemoglobin level after the first 12–24 months of therapy.
- Maintain platelet count of ≥100,000/mm^3.
- Reduce bleeding tendency due to low platelet count, platelet abnormality, or coagulation defects.
- Prevent osteopenia, osteoporosis, bone pain, and bone complications.
- Improve mobility and physical activity [1, 2].

6.3 Choice of Treatment for GD

Treatment options for Gaucher disease, depending on disease severity, type, and initial assessment, include enzyme replacement (ERT), substrate reduction (SRT), gene therapy (GT), hematopoietic cell transplantation, splenectomy, and enzyme enhancement therapy (EET) (Fig. 6.1).

6.3.1 Enzyme Replacement Therapy (ERT)

The Guidelines for ERT in children and adults with GD, developed by a consensus of international experts using data acquired from the International Collaborative Gaucher Group (ICGG) Gaucher Registry and local experience, recommended the following indications for ERT:

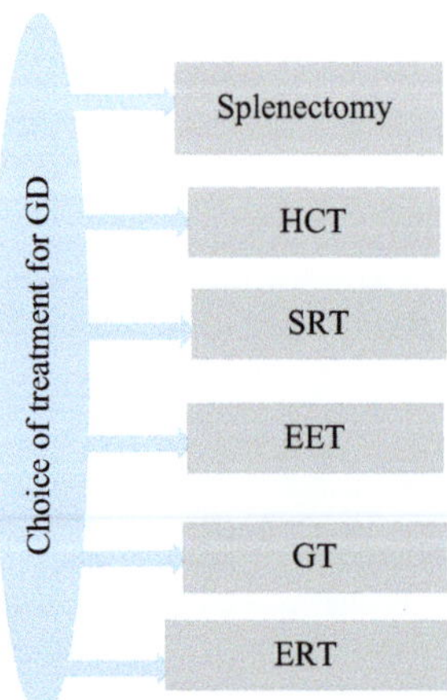

Fig. 6.1 Choice of treatment in ERT

- **Recommended Indication for Nonneuronopathic GD1.**
  Children: symptomatic children with.
  - Visceromegaly.
  - Anemia.
  - Thrombocytopenia.
  - Malnutrition.
  - Growth retardation.
  - Impaired development.
  - Fatigue.

  Adults: symptomatic adults with.
  - Anemia.
  - Thrombocytopenia less than 60,000/microliter.
  - Liver size more than 2.5 times.
  - Spleen size more than 15 times.
  - Skeletal disease (radiologic or clinical evidence) [3–5].
- **Recommended Indication in Neuronopathic GD**
  Patients with chronic neuronopathic GD3.
  Siblings of patients with chronic neuronopathic GD who are proven to have GD.
  Patients with the following high-risk genotypes: L444P/L444P (c.1448 T > C homozygote), D409H/D409H (c.1342G > C homozygote), and L444P/D409H (c.1448 T > C/c.1342G > C heterozygote).
  Onset of severe systemic GD at ≤2 years of age [6, 7].
  GD3 disease with visceromegaly.
  Patients who are suspected to have GD3 (according to the genotype and family history) before the onset of neurologic signs or symptoms [8, 9].
  ERT may be used as a palliative treatment in GD2 diseases with visceral manifestations without improvement of neurologic symptoms and outcome [10, 11].

Recombinant enzymes can overcome blocks in the catabolic pathway, enhancing the clearance rate of stored substrate. These enzymes are deglycosylated and expose their mannose residues, allowing macrophage receptors to uptake them for transfer to lysosomes. Notable recombinant glucocerebrosidase used in ERT for GD includes

- Imiglucerase produced using mammalian cells (Cerezyme®, Sanofi-Genzyme, and Abcertin®, ISU Abxis).
- Velaglucerase alfa produced using human fibroblasts (Vpriv®, Shire, authorized in 2010).
- Taliglucerase alfa produced using carrot cells (Elelyso®, Pfizer; not approved for use in the European Union) [12].

Imiglucerase is a recombinant protein produced by genetically engineered CHO cells, resembling human glucocerebrosidase with a single amino acid substitution: arginine is replaced by histidine at position 495 [13, 14] (Fig. 6.2).

- **Administration of ERT**

Initial enzyme doses should be based on age, weight at referral, molecular status, and disease severity [2]. For children and at-risk adults with GD1, the standard starting dose is 60 units/kg, given intravenously every 2 weeks over 1–2 h [15].

The minimum starting dose for children is 30 units/kg biweekly when drug availability is

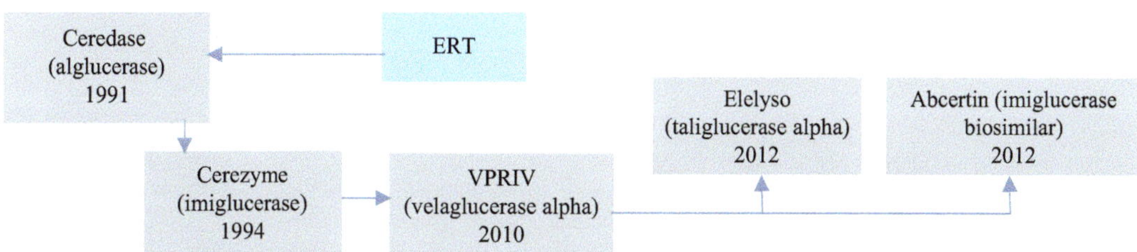

Fig. 6.2 Algorithm of developing ERT over time

limited. If treatment goals are unmet, the enzyme dose should be increased [3, 16].

The treatment approach and follow-up for newly diagnosed adult and child patients with GD1 are shown in Fig. 6.3 and Fig. 6.4, respectively.

Measuring the weight and adjusting the enzyme dose before every injection is essential. For adult patients with severe conditions, such as life-threatening hepatopulmonary syndrome and pulmonary hypertension, immediate intervention is crucial, which is why the initial dose of imiglucerase is typically 120 U/kg body weight every 2 weeks. Once symptoms improve, the enzyme dose can be reduced to a maintenance regimen [17].

After achieving the therapeutic goals, the dose may be reduced, but not less than 30 U/kg, to prevent relapse in skeletal involvement during long-term maintenance therapy. A low dose of imiglucerase (around 10 U/kg/every 2 weeks) has improved anemia and thrombocytopenia associated with Gaucher disease and may be considered in a resource-limited setting when other options are unavailable [18]. Enzyme dosage should be adjusted on the individual clinical course and biomarkers:

- Increase the dose by 50% if bone crises persist [19].
- If symptoms such as anemia, thrombocytopenia, visceromegaly, and disease biomarkers do not improve after 6 months, a dose increase may be necessary. However, further evaluation is required for patients who do not meet their therapeutic goals within 3–6 months before considering this change [16].
- After meeting all therapeutic goals, a dose reduction is permissible [2]. Protocols using low doses of 15–30 U/kg/month, administered in thrice weekly doses, have shown good outcomes and are suitable for patients with stable disease [20, 21].

Treatment should be lifelong as there is a risk of relapse or disease progression with prolonged interruptions [2].

– **Effectiveness of ERT**

Studies indicate that all ERTs exhibit comparable efficacy [22–24]. There are currently no guidelines favoring imiglucerase over velaglucerase or any other enzyme for treating Gaucher disease type 1, although the availability of the enzyme in each country is a key factor. Imiglucerase is the sole enzyme approved for GD3, and no enzymes are indicated for GD2 treatment [25, 26].

The recombinant enzyme cannot cross the blood-brain barrier and has a limited effect on

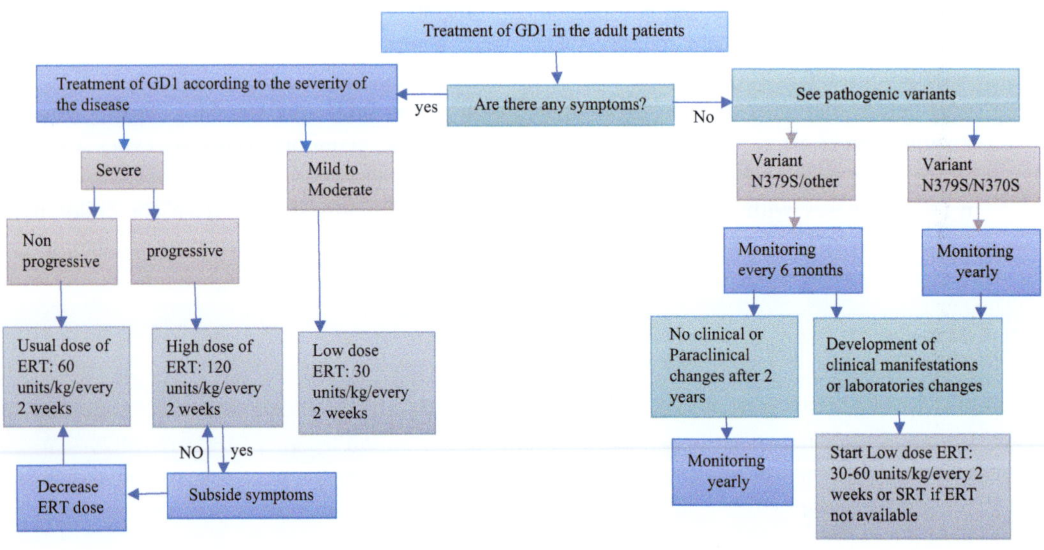

Fig. 6.3 Approach to treatment and follow-up for newly diagnosed adult patients with GD type 1

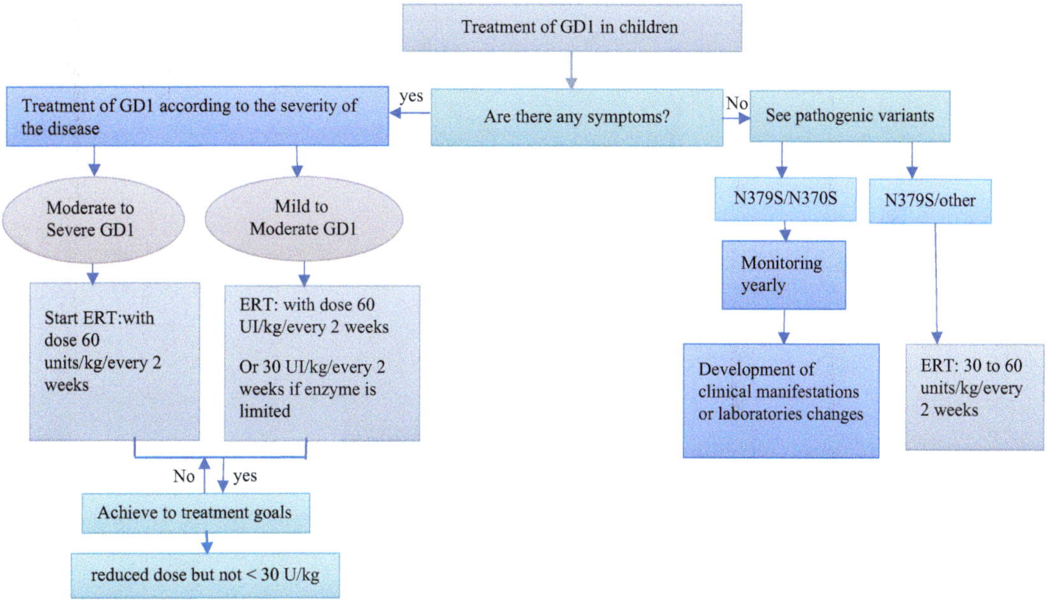

Fig. 6.4 Approach to treatment and follow-up for newly diagnosed children patients with GD type 1

neurological diseases. Consequently, ERT is primarily used to reduce liver and spleen volume and improve hematologic disorders (such as hemoglobin levels and platelet count), but it does not alleviate neurological symptoms in GD2 and GD3 [27]. Response to ERT varies among patients with GD1, and its effectiveness includes (Fig. 6.5) the following:

Liver and spleen volumes decrease by 20–30% within 1–2 years of treatment, with reductions by 30–40% after 5 years. In some cases, spleen size may remain over five times normal [28].

A significant increase in platelet counts in thrombocytopenic patients with an intact spleen is observed within 2 years and can be maintained for up to 5 years [28].

However, the increase in platelet counts is less pronounced in those with severe baseline thrombocytopenia. After 4–5 years of therapy, 25% of patients exhibit mild thrombocytopenia (platelet count 120 × 109/L), while 2% have severe thrombocytopenia (platelet count 60 × 109/L) [29].

Low baseline platelet counts and larger baseline splenic diameters are predictors of persistent thrombocytopenia.

Conversely, in some splenectomized patients, platelet counts may normalize within 6–12 months if thrombocytopenia is due to bone marrow failure [28].

Normal or near-normal hemoglobin levels are typically reached within 6–12 months of treatment, and the response to ERT may continue for up to 5 years [28].

Skeletal disorder may improve after 2–3 years of therapy [3], with the most significant gains in BMD seen in younger patients [30].

Regular monitoring of bone mineral density through dual-energy X-ray absorptiometry (DXA) and marrow infiltration via magnetic resonance imaging (MRI) is recommended [31].

Biomarker levels, including macrophage activation (chitotriosidase or CCL18), angiotensin-converting enzyme (ACE), and glucosylsphingosine (lyso-Gb1) return to near-normal values with enzyme replacement [32, 33].

ERT can decrease polyclonal hypergammaglobulinemia but has little effect on monoclonal gammopathy [7].

Fatigue reduction is anticipated within 6 months of starting ERT [34].

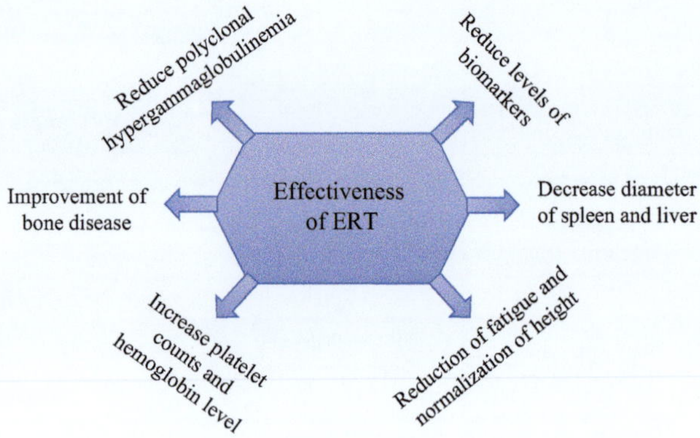

Fig. 6.5 Effectiveness and response algorithm to ERT

Long-term ERT promotes increased height velocity in children with GD [35].

Children with GD who begin ERT in their first decade experience normal puberty onset, while those who do not receive ERT have delayed puberty [36, 37].

– **ERT During Pregnancy**

Velaglucerase or imiglucerase treatment can reduce Gaucher-related complications in pregnant women with GD without causing fetal malformations. Additionally, ERT can raise platelet counts, which is crucial for delivery and the postpartum period [38–41].

– **ERT Adverse Effects**

ERT is a safe and effective treatment for GD. While immunological immunoglobulin E (IgE)-independent reactions such as flu-like symptoms, along with some acute IgE-mediated reactions like pruritus, urticaria, angioedema, flushing, respiratory symptoms, and hypotension, are rare, they can occur during the intravenous infusion of ERT.

These reactions may be mitigated by reducing the infusion rate or administering antihistamines and glucocorticoids [3, 42]. The risk of allergic reactions appears to be slightly higher and more common with taliglucerase [39].

A concern with ERT is the potential formation of antibodies against the enzyme, which occurs in 10–15% of patients treated with imiglucerase, 1% with velaglucerase, and 22% with taliglucerase.

However, routine monitoring for IgG antibodies is not recommended due to the rarity of this occurrence [43].

– **Monitoring ERT**

To evaluate treatment response and adjust enzyme dosage, a regular monitoring schedule is essential for patient assessment.

The International Collaborative Gaucher Group (ICGG) offers valuable recommendations for the optimal management of patients with GD (Table 6.1) [5, 44].

Additional tests should include vitamin B12, iron, ferritin, iron-binding capacity, prothrombin time, white blood count, activated partial thromboplastin time, hepatitis profile, aspartate aminotransferase, alanine aminotransferase, alkaline phosphatase, phosphorous, calcium, albumin, total protein, total/direct bilirubin, and serum immunoelectrophoresis—all measured according to the patient's age and disease state.

6.3.2 Substrate Reduction Therapy (SRT)

Substrate reduction therapy, proposed by Radin et al. in 1972 [45], received Food and Drug Administration (FDA) approval for the treatment of GD in 2003.

SRT reduces glycolipid accumulation by inhibiting glucocerebroside synthesis, offering a

Table 6.1 Monitoring recommendations for patients with Gaucher disease type 1 [5, 44]

Parameters	Frequency			
	Receiving ERT, has not achieved the goal	Receiving ERT, has achieved the goal	Asymptomatic not receiving enzyme therapy	At the time of dose change or significant clinical complication
[a]Spleen and liver diameters	Every 12–24 months	[f]Every 12–24 months	Every 12–24 months	Should be checked
MRI spine (sagittal T1 weighted) (only in children) MRI femora (coronal T1 and T2 weighted)	Every 12 months	Every 12–24 months	Every 24 months or less frequently if consistently normal	Should be checked (in symptomatic patients)
Plain radiographs [b]Children: Pelvis, long bones, spine [c]Adults: Lateral spine; AP of entire femoral	Every 12 months	Every 12–24 months	Every 12–24 months	Should be checked (in symptomatic patients)
[d]DXA spine and hips	Every 12 months	Every 12–24 months	Every 12–24 monthsin adults	–
Hemoglobin	Every 3–6 months	Every 12–24 months	Every 12 months	Should be checked
Platelets	Every 3–6 months	Every 12–24 months	Every 12 months	Should be checked
Chitotriosidase, PARC/CCL18, HDL	Every 3–6 months	Every 12–24 months	Every 12 months	Should be checked
Antibody	Optional sample after 6 months of therapy (if indicated)	–	–	–
Serum immunoelectrophoresis (only in adults)	Every 12–24 months in patients >50 years	Every 12–24 months	Every 12–24 months in patients >50 years	Should be checked
Cardiopulmonary Children Forced vital capacity Peak expiratory flow rate High-resolution chest computed tomography Echocardiography Electrocardiogram	Repeat if abnormal at baseline or if symptoms develop	Every 12–24 months	Repeat if abnormal at aseline or if symptoms develop	Should be checked (in symptomatic patients)
Cardiopulmonary Adults Electrocardiogram Chest radiograph Doppler echocardiogram	Annual evaluation if signs/symptoms of Cardiopulmonary disease is present	Every 12–24 months	Every 12–24 months for those with borderline or above normal pulmonary pressures at baseline	Should be checked (in symptomatic patients)
[e]Quality of life, SF-36d, PedsQL, or KidscreenR (179,180)	Every 12 months	Every 12–24 months	Every 12 months	Should be checked
Pain assessment	Every 6 months	Every 12–24 months	Every 12 months	Should be checked

(continued)

Table 6.1 (continued)

Parameters	Frequency: Receiving ERT, has not achieved the goal	Receiving ERT, has achieved the goal	Asymptomatic not receiving enzyme therapy	At the time of dose change or significant clinical complication
Measure of weight and height	Every 6 months	Every 12–24 months	Every 12 months	Should be checked

All parameters that are normal at baseline do not need follow-up within 6 months

[a]Spleen and liver diameters should be measured by MRI, but ultrasonography can be used if MRI is not available

[b]Plain radiographs of the spine are only recommended if the patient is symptomatic or has severe disease, poor growth, or skeletal deformity (kyphosis)

[c]If the patient is symptomatic

[d]Annually until normal, then every 3 years in treated patients. BMD should be compared with normal data for age and gender

[e]The Short-Form 36 (SF-36) Health Survey is of limited value in very young patients

[f]Ultrasound exams are preferred for monitoring visceromegaly in asymptomatic children

potential alternative to ERT for certain patients [46–52] (Fig. 6.6).

Eliglustat and miglustat are orally administered, quickly diffusing throughout tissues, and have the potential advantage of improving bone involvement through direct drug delivery to bone compartments [53].

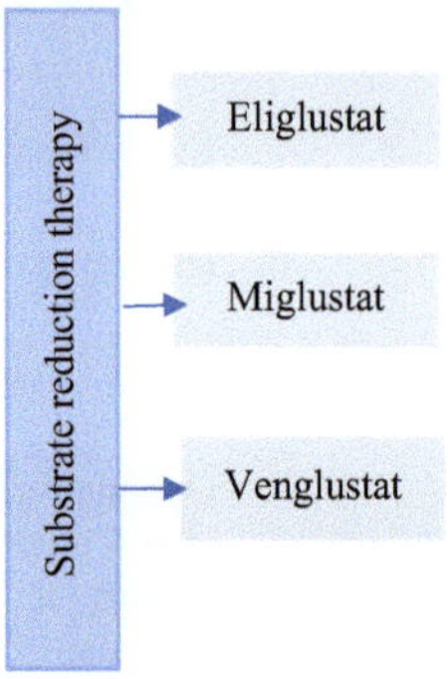

Fig. 6.6 Substrate reduction therapy

- **Miglustat**

  Miglustat (Zavesca®, Actelion) is a GlcCer synthase inhibitor that reduces GlcCer biosynthesis in Gaucher cells. It has been available in European countries since November 2002 for treating mild to moderate GD1, and it is approved in the United States when ERT is unsuitable.

  This treatment is not approved in children with GD1 but may help reduce seizure frequency in those with GD3 [54].

  Some studies indicate that miglustat treatment can reduce liver and spleen volume within 6–18 months, improve clinical symptoms over 2 years, and lower chitotriosidase levels, although its efficacy on hematological parameters is limited [55].

  It has been used as maintenance therapy for a patient who achieved treatment goals with ERT.

  The common side effects of miglustat include diarrhea, weight loss, tremors, and peripheral neuropathy, which may improve with dietary changes or antidiarrheal medications [56].

  The recommended dosage is 100 mg orally three times a day, with a possible reduction to 100 mg once or twice daily for patients experiencing adverse effects [57]. Miglustat is contraindicated during pregnancy.

- **Eliglustat**

  Eliglustat (Cerdelga™, Sanofi/Genzyme), a widely used SRT, received European Union approval in 2015 and US approval in 2014. As an analog of ceramide, it is more specific and potent than miglustat [58].

  Before starting eliglustat, patients should undergo a CYP2D6 status assessment to determine their metabolizer classification (extensive, intermediate, or poor) because Eliglustat is eliminated through the CYP2D6 pathway.

  The dose for extensive and intermediate metabolizers is 84 mg orally twice daily, and for poor metabolizers, it is 84 mg once daily [59].

Eliglustat is ineffective for CYP2D6 ultrarapid metabolizers as it does not achieve sufficient plasma concentrations.

Eliglustat is contraindicated in patients with preexisting cardiac disease, those taking class 1A and class III antiarrhythmics, and individuals with galactose intolerance, lactase deficiency, or glucose-galactose malabsorption [60].

Concomitant use of CYP2D6 and CYP3A inhibitors is contraindicated, and it is not approved in pregnancy.

A clinical trial of eliglustat in pediatric patients with GD1 or GD3 is in progress (NCT03485677).

– **Venglustat**

  Venglustat as an SRT can penetrate the brain, and it is currently undergoing clinical trials for adults with GD3 (NCT02843035 venglustat).

  Venglustat prevents the conversion of ceramide to glucosylceramide, thereby decreasing the substrate available for glycosphingolipid synthesis [61].

6.3.3 Splenectomy

ERT has minimized the need for splenectomy, which is related to bone outcome and subsequent episodes of avascular necrosis [62]. There are a few indications for splenectomy, including

Life-threatening thrombocytopenia unresponsive to ERT.
High bleeding risk.
Severe abdominal discomfort due to recurrent splenic infarction.
Inferior vena cava syndrome.
Severe restrictive pulmonary disease.
Lack of access to ERT or SRT [63].

6.3.4 Hematopoietic Stem Cell Transplantation

ERT is a safe and effective treatment for GD with minimal side effects.

While HSCT can potentially cure GD, its safety and efficacy remain unassessed due to limited experience.

Additionally, there are no definitive guidelines recommending HSCT for GD. Hence, HSCT should be considered only for select patients, particularly those with GD3 presenting before neurological symptoms appear [64, 65].

6.3.5 Gene Therapy

Gene therapy is an emerging definitive treatment for GD, with two types of vectors under development: adeno-associated vectors (AAVs) and integrating lentiviruses.

Both methods aim to achieve sustained transgene expression in cells. Three clinical trials are underway: neuropathic GD (NCT04411654) with AAV9 gene therapy, GD1 (NCT04145037) using lentiviral-based, and GD1 (NCT05324943) employing liver-targeted AAV gene therapy.

6.3.6 Enzyme Enhancement Therapy (EET)

EET as pharmacologic chaperones can enhance the residual activity of mutant glucocerebrosidase by stabilizing its folding and reducing enzyme degradation, offering a potential future therapy for GD [9, 66, 67].

- **Isofagomine**

  Amicus developed isofagomine, a small molecule chaperone that stabilizes misfolded p. Asn409Ser GCase and enhances enzymatic function in vitro in patient fibroblasts [68]. However, clinical trials demonstrated poor cellular uptake and no clinical improvement [69].

6.3.7 Noninhibitory Chaperone

- **Ambroxol**

High-dose oral ambroxol, used as a noninhibitory chaperone alongside ERT, could significantly enhance lymphocyte glucocerebrosidase activity and lower glucosylsphingosine levels in the cerebrospinal fluid of patients with neuronopathic GD.

Neurologic symptoms, including myoclonic epilepsy and pupillary light reflex dysfunction, improved in all patients [70]. One study reported improved or stable neurologic symptoms, reduced fatigue, and increased physical activity with ambroxol at a median dose of 435 mg/day [71]. Ambroxol was initially administered at 10 mg/kg/day for 6 months, then increased to 15 mg/kg/day for 2.5 years, resulting in bilateral remodeling of the femoral head's sphericity [72].

- **Arimoclomol**

Arimoclomol is another noninhibitory chaperone that enhances HSP70 levels, facilitating the folding and maturation of mutant glucocerebrosidase in the cells and a neuronal model of GD [73].

- **Histone Deacetylase Inhibitors**

Histone deacetylase inhibitors (HDACIs) may be effective in treating potential GD and other protein-misfolding diseases, including Huntington's disease, Niemann-Pick type C disease, and cystic fibrosis. HDACI, such as suberoylanilide hydroxamic acid (SAHA), could increase GCase activity in fibroblasts from patients with GD1 and GD2 by modulating two molecular chaperones: heat-shock protein (Hsp) 90 and Hsp 70 [67].

- **Other Noninhibitory Chaperone Agents**
  The lead molecule NCGC758 enhanced GCase activity, reversed lipid storage in patient-derived induced pluripotent stem cell (iPSC) macrophages, and restored their impaired function [74].

  NCGC607 has been shown to boost GCase activity and reverse lipid storage in patient-derived iPSC-dopaminergic neurons [75].

  The small molecule modulator S-181 may enhance β-glucocerebrosidase function in both mutant and wild-type forms in an iPSC-dopaminergic model with the c.84insG mutation and in a murine model [76].

6.3.8 Supportive Care

Supportive care is an important part of the management of patients with GD, especially in children.

- **Bone Diseases**
  Severe bone crises respond to intravenous fluids and and analgesics, particularly nonsteroidal anti-inflammatory drugs and acetaminophen [16].

  Nonsteroidal anti-inflammatory drugs should be avoided in individuals with moderate-to-severe thrombocytopenia.

  Narcotics can be administered for severe crises that do not respond to analgesics. Another option for severe and intolerable pain is oral prednisolone at a dosage of 20 mg/m^2 per day [77].

  Osteomyelitis should be considered during bone crisis and pain episodes. The early diagnosis and management of osteomyelitis are linked to fewer complications and reduced morbidity. Laboratory and imaging studies, including blood cultures, erythrocyte sedimentation rate (ESR), C-reactive protein (CRP), radionuclide scans, magnetic resonance imaging, and bone biopsies/cultures, may be necessary to confirm bone involvement [9].

  Osteopenia in adults with GD can improve with ERT, though it may occasionally be resistant. In this condition, bisphosphonates like alendronate, along with calcium and vitamin D supplements, should be considered [78].

Orthopedic procedures, like joint replacement, may be necessary.

Despite comprehensive supportive care for bone involvement [79].

- **Bleeding Tendency**
  Patients with GD face the risk of bleeding from thrombocytopenia, impaired platelet function, and coagulation factors. Thus, a hematologist assessment is essential before a major surgery or dental procedure or during pregnancy and childbirth. Proper evaluation and preparation are necessary before these procedures [2].
- **Severe Anemia**
  Blood transfusion should be considered for severe anemia and/or bleeding diathesis unresponsive to ERT [80].

References

1. Biegstraaten M, Cox TM, Belmatoug N, Berger MG, Collin-Histed T, Vom Dahl S, et al. Management goals for type 1 Gaucher disease: AN expert consensus document from the European working group on Gaucher disease. Blood Cells Mol Dis. 2018;68:203–8.
2. Pastores GM, Weinreb NJ, Aerts H, Andria G, Cox TM, Giralt M, et al. Therapeutic goals in the treatment of Gaucher disease. Semin Hematol. 2004;41(4 Suppl 5):4–14.
3. Charrow J, Andersson HC, Kaplan P, Kolodny EH, Mistry P, Pastores G, et al. Enzyme replacement therapy and monitoring for children with type 1 Gaucher disease: consensus recommendations. J Pediatr. 2004;144(1):112–20.
4. Grabowski GA, Andria G, Baldellou A, Campbell PE, Charrow J, Cohen IJ, et al. Pediatric non-neuronopathic Gaucher disease: presentation, diagnosis and assessment. Consensus statements. Eur J Pediatr. 2004;163(2):58–66.
5. Weinreb NJ, Aggio MC, Andersson HC, Andria G, Charrow J, Clarke JT, et al. Gaucher disease type 1: revised recommendations on evaluations and monitoring for adult patients. Semin Hematol. 2004;41(4 Suppl 5):15–22.
6. Vellodi A, Bembi B, de Villemeur TB, Collin-Histed T, Erikson A, Mengel E, et al. Management of neuronopathic Gaucher disease: a European consensus. J Inherit Metab Dis. 2001;24(3):319–27.
7. Vellodi A, Tylki-Szymanska A, Davies EH, Kolodny E, Bembi B, Collin-Histed T, et al. Management of neuronopathic Gaucher disease: revised recommendations. J Inherit Metab Dis. 2009;32(5):660–4.
8. Grabowski GA. Recent clinical progress in Gaucher disease. Curr Opin Pediatr. 2005;17(4):519–24.
9. Jmoudiak M, Futerman AH. Gaucher disease: pathological mechanisms and modern management. Br J Haematol. 2005;129(2):178–88.
10. Prows CA, Sanchez N, Daugherty C, Grabowski GA. Gaucher disease: enzyme therapy in the acute neuronopathic variant. Am J Med Genet. 1997;71(1):16–21.
11. Roshan Lal T, Seehra GK, Steward AM, Poffenberger CN, Ryan E, Tayebi N, et al. The natural history of type 2 Gaucher disease in the 21st century: a retrospective study. Neurology. 2020;95(15):e2119–e30.
12. Stirnemann J, Belmatoug N, Camou F, Serratrice C, Froissart R, Caillaud C, et al. A review of Gaucher disease pathophysiology, clinical presentation and treatments. Int J Mol Sci. 2017;18(2)
13. Choi JH, Lee BH, Ko JM, Sohn YB, Lee JS, Kim GH, et al. A phase 2 multi-center, open-label, switch-over trial to evaluate the safety and efficacy of Abcertin® in patients with type 1 Gaucher disease. J Korean Med Sci. 2015;30(4):378–84.
14. Lee BH, Abdalla AF, Choi JH, Beshlawy AE, Kim GH, Heo SH, et al. A multicenter, open-label, phase III study of Abcertin in Gaucher disease. Medicine (Baltimore). 2017;96(45):e8492.
15. Andersson HC, Charrow J, Kaplan P, Mistry P, Pastores GM, Prakash-Cheng A, et al. Individualization of long-term enzyme replacement therapy for Gaucher disease. Genet Med. 2005;7(2):105–10.
16. Kaplan P, Baris H, De Meirleir L, Di Rocco M, El-Beshlawy A, Huemer M, et al. Revised recommendations for the management of Gaucher disease in children. Eur J Pediatr. 2013;172(4):447–58.
17. Mistry PK, Sirrs S, Chan A, Pritzker MR, Duffy TP, Grace ME, et al. Pulmonary hypertension in type 1 Gaucher's disease: genetic and epigenetic determinants of phenotype and response to therapy. Mol Genet Metab. 2002;77(1–2):91–8.
18. Heitner R, Arndt S, Levin JB. Imiglucerase low-dose therapy for paediatric Gaucher disease–a long-term cohort study. S Afr Med J 2004;94(8):647–651.
19. Cohen IJ, Katz K, Kornreich L, Horev G, Frish A, Zaizov R. Low-dose high-frequency enzyme replacement therapy prevents fractures without complete suppression of painful bone crises in patients with severe juvenile onset type I Gaucher disease. Blood Cells Mol Dis. 1998;24(3):296–302.
20. Beutler E, Nguyen NJ, Henneberger MW, Smolec JM, McPherson RA, West C, et al. Gaucher disease: gene frequencies in the Ashkenazi Jewish population. Am J Hum Genet. 1993;52(1):85–8.
21. Zimran A, Hadas-Halpern I, Zevin S, Levy-Lahad E, Abrahamov A. Low-dose high-frequency enzyme replacement therapy for very young children with severe Gaucher disease. Br J Haematol. 1993;85(4):783–6.
22. Aviezer D, Brill-Almon E, Shaaltiel Y, Hashmueli S, Bartfeld D, Mizrachi S, et al. A plant-derived recombinant human glucocerebrosidase enzyme–

a preclinical and phase I investigation. PLoS One. 2009;4(3):e4792.
23. Pastores GM, Rosenbloom B, Weinreb N, Goker-Alpan O, Grabowski G, Cohn GM, et al. A multicenter open-label treatment protocol (HGT-GCB-058) of velaglucerase alfa enzyme replacement therapy in patients with Gaucher disease type 1: safety and tolerability. Genet Med. 2014;16(5):359–66.
24. Zimran A, Brill-Almon E, Chertkoff R, Petakov M, Blanco-Favela F, Muñoz ET, et al. Pivotal trial with plant cell-expressed recombinant glucocerebrosidase, taliglucerase alfa, a novel enzyme replacement therapy for Gaucher disease. Blood. 2011;118(22):5767–73.
25. Mignot C, Doummar D, Maire I, De Villemeur TB. Type 2 Gaucher disease: 15 new cases and review of the literature. Brain Dev. 2006;28(1):39–48.
26. Weiss K, Gonzalez A, Lopez G, Pedoeim L, Groden C, Sidransky E. The clinical management of type 2 Gaucher disease. Mol Genet Metab. 2015;114(2):110–22.
27. Altarescu G, Hill S, Wiggs E, Jeffries N, Kreps C, Parker CC, et al. The efficacy of enzyme replacement therapy in patients with chronic neuronopathic Gaucher's disease. J Pediatr. 2001;138(4):539–47.
28. Weinreb NJ, Charrow J, Andersson HC, Kaplan P, Kolodny EH, Mistry P, et al. Effectiveness of enzyme replacement therapy in 1028 patients with type 1 Gaucher disease after 2 to 5 years of treatment: a report from the Gaucher registry. Am J Med. 2002;113(2):112–9.
29. Hollak CE, Belmatoug N, Cole JA, Vom Dahl S, Deegan PB, Goldblatt J, et al. Characteristics of type I Gaucher disease associated with persistent thrombocytopenia after treatment with imiglucerase for 4-5 years. Br J Haematol. 2012;158(4):528–38.
30. Mistry PK, Weinreb NJ, Kaplan P, Cole JA, Gwosdow AR, Hangartner T. Osteopenia in Gaucher disease develops early in life: response to imiglucerase enzyme therapy in children, adolescents and adults. Blood Cells Mol Dis. 2011;46(1):66–72.
31. Hughes D, Mikosch P, Belmatoug N, Carubbi F, Cox T, Goker-Alpan O, et al. Gaucher disease in bone: from pathophysiology to practice. J Bone Miner Res. 2019;34(6):996–1013.
32. Dekker N, van Dussen L, Hollak CE, Overkleeft H, Scheij S, Ghauharali K, et al. Elevated plasma glucosylsphingosine in Gaucher disease: relation to phenotype, storage cell markers, and therapeutic response. Blood. 2011;118(16):e118–27.
33. Hurvitz N, Dinur T, Becker-Cohen M, Cozma C, Hovakimyan M, Oppermann S, et al. Glucosylsphingosine (lyso-Gb1) as a biomarker for monitoring treated and untreated children with Gaucher disease. Int J Mol Sci. 2019;20(12)
34. Beutler E. Enzyme replacement therapy for Gaucher's disease. Baillieres Clin Haematol. 1997;10(4):751–63.
35. Andersson H, Kaplan P, Kacena K, Yee J. Eight-year clinical outcomes of long-term enzyme replacement therapy for 884 children with Gaucher disease type 1. Pediatrics. 2008;122(6):1182–90.
36. González DC, Ruiz A, Oliveri B. Osteomalacia as an extraintestinal manifestation of celiac disease in a patient treated for Gaucher disease. Endocr Metab Sci. 2020;1(1):100052.
37. Kaplan P, Mazur A, Manor O, Charrow J, Esplin J, Gribble TJ, et al. Acceleration of retarded growth in children with Gaucher disease after treatment with alglucerase. J Pediatr. 1996;129(1):149–53.
38. Cohen Y, Frydman D, Rotem R, Kofman R, Zimran A, Revel-Vilk S, et al. Risk of postpartum hemorrhage in multiparous women with Gaucher disease: a call for reconsidering enzyme replacement therapy in all pregnant patients. J Inherit Metab Dis. 2021;44(5):1165–73.
39. Elstein D, Hughes D, Goker-Alpan O, Stivel M, Baris HN, Cohen IJ, et al. Outcome of pregnancies in women receiving velaglucerase alfa for Gaucher disease. J Obstet Gynaecol Res. 2014;40(4):968–75.
40. Lau H, Belmatoug N, Deegan P, Goker-Alpan O, Schwartz IVD, Shankar SP, et al. Reported outcomes of 453 pregnancies in patients with Gaucher disease: an analysis from the Gaucher outcome survey. Blood Cells Mol Dis. 2018;68:226–31.
41. Zimran A, Morris E, Mengel E, Kaplan P, Belmatoug N, Hughes DA, et al. The female Gaucher patient: the impact of enzyme replacement therapy around key reproductive events (menstruation, pregnancy and menopause). Blood Cells Mol Dis. 2009;43(3):264–88.
42. Pastores GM. Recombinant glucocerebrosidase (imiglucerase) as a therapy for Gaucher disease. BioDrugs. 2010;24(1):41–7.
43. Pastores GM, Shankar SP, Petakov M, Giraldo P, Rosenbaum H, Amato DJ, et al. Enzyme replacement therapy with taliglucerase alfa: 36-month safety and efficacy results in adult patients with Gaucher disease previously treated with imiglucerase. Am J Hematol. 2016;91(7):661–5.
44. Sanofi Genzyme Rare Disease Registries [Internet]. August 03, 2022. https://www.registrynxt.com.
45. Radin NS, Arora RC, Ullman MD, Brenkert AL, Austin J. A possible therapeutic approach to Krabbe's globoid leukodystrophy and the status of cerebroside synthesis in the disorder. Res Commun Chem Pathol Pharmacol. 1972;3(3):637–44.
46. Beutler E, Saven A. Misuse of marrow examination in the diagnosis of Gaucher disease. Blood. 1990;76(3):646–8.
47. Kenet G, Hayek S, Mor M, Lubetsky A, Miller L, Rosenberg N, et al. The 1226G (N370S) Gaucher mutation among patients with Legg-Calve-Perthes disease. Blood Cells Mol Dis. 2003;31(1):72–4.
48. Kooper AJ, Janssens PM, de Groot AN, Liebrand-van Sambeek ML, van den Berg CJ, Tan-Sindhunata GB, et al. Lysosomal storage diseases in non-immune hydrops fetalis pregnancies. Clin Chim Acta. 2006;371(1–2):176–82.
49. Srivastava P, Srivastava A, Srivastava P, Betigeri AV, Verma M. Congenital ichthyosis – collodion baby case report. J Clin Diagn Res. 2016;10(6):Sj01-2.

50. Stewart AJ, Jones RD. Pseudo-Gaucher cells in myelodysplasia. J Clin Pathol. 1999;52(12):917–8.
51. Tayebi N, Lopez G, Do J, Sidransky E, Pro-cathepsin D. Prosaposin, and progranulin: lysosomal networks in parkinsonism. Trends Mol Med. 2020;26(10):913–23.
52. Turner BM, Hirschhorn K. Properties of beta-glucosidase in cultured skin fibroblasts from controls and patients with Gaucher disease. Am J Hum Genet. 1978;30(4):346–58.
53. Limgala RP, Goker-Alpan O. Effect of substrate reduction therapy in comparison to enzyme replacement therapy on immune aspects and bone involvement in Gaucher disease. Biomol Ther. 2020;10(4)
54. Kraoua I, Sedel F, Caillaud C, Froissart R, Stirnemann J, Chaurand G, et al. A French experience of type 3 Gaucher disease: phenotypic diversity and neurological outcome of 10 patients. Brain Dev. 2011;33(2):131–9.
55. Pastores GM, Barnett NL, Kolodny EH. An open-label, noncomparative study of miglustat in type I Gaucher disease: efficacy and tolerability over 24 months of treatment. Clin Ther. 2005;27(8):1215–27.
56. Cox T, Lachmann R, Hollak C, Aerts J, van Weely S, Hrebícek M, et al. Novel oral treatment of Gaucher's disease with N-butyldeoxynojirimycin (OGT 918) to decrease substrate biosynthesis. Lancet. 2000;355(9214):1481–5.
57. Heitner R, Elstein D, Aerts J, Weely S, Zimran A. Low-dose N-butyldeoxynojirimycin (OGT 918) for type I Gaucher disease. Blood Cells Mol Dis. 2002;28(2):127–33.
58. Cox TM, Drelichman G, Cravo R, Balwani M, Burrow TA, Martins AM, et al. Eliglustat compared with imiglucerase in patients with Gaucher's disease type 1 stabilised on enzyme replacement therapy: a phase 3, randomised, open-label, non-inferiority trial. Lancet. 2015;385(9985):2355–62.
59. Balwani M, Burrow TA, Charrow J, Goker-Alpan O, Kaplan P, Kishnani PS, et al. Recommendations for the use of eliglustat in the treatment of adults with Gaucher disease type 1 in the United States. Mol Genet Metab. 2016;117(2):95–103.
60. Belmatoug N, Di Rocco M, Fraga C, Giraldo P, Hughes D, Lukina E, et al. Management and monitoring recommendations for the use of eliglustat in adults with type 1 Gaucher disease in Europe. Eur J Intern Med. 2017;37:25–32.
61. Deegan PB, Goker-Alpan O, Geberhiwot T, Hopkin RJ, Lukina E, Tylki-Szymanska A, et al. Venglustat, an orally administered glucosylceramide synthase inhibitor: assessment over 3 years in adult males with classic Fabry disease in an open-label phase 2 study and its extension study. Mol Genet Metab. 2023;138(2):106963.
62. Deegan PB, Pavlova E, Tindall J, Stein PE, Bearcroft P, Mehta A, et al. Osseous manifestations of adult Gaucher disease in the era of enzyme replacement therapy. Medicine (Baltimore). 2011;90(1):52–60.
63. Zimran A, Elstein D, Schiffmann R, Abrahamov A, Goldberg M, Bar-Maor JA, et al. Outcome of partial splenectomy for type I Gaucher disease. J Pediatr. 1995;126(4):596–7.
64. Chavananon S, Sripornsawan P, Songthawee N, Chotsampancharoen T. Successful treatment of Gaucher disease with matched sibling hematopoietic stem cell transplantation: a case report and literature review. J Pediatr Hematol Oncol. 2021;43(8):e1153–e5.
65. Ito S, Barrett AJ. Gauchers disease–a reappraisal of hematopoietic stem cell transplantation. Pediatr Hematol Oncol 2013;30(2):61–70.
66. Khanna R, Benjamin ER, Pellegrino L, Schilling A, Rigat BA, Soska R, et al. The pharmacological chaperone isofagomine increases the activity of the Gaucher disease L444P mutant form of beta-glucosidase. FEBS J. 2010;277(7):1618–38.
67. Lu J, Yang C, Chen M, Ye DY, Lonser RR, Brady RO, et al. Histone deacetylase inhibitors prevent the degradation and restore the activity of glucocerebrosidase in Gaucher disease. Proc Natl Acad Sci USA. 2011;108(52):21200–5.
68. Steet RA, Chung S, Wustman B, Powe A, Do H, Kornfeld SA. The iminosugar isofagomine increases the activity of N370S mutant acid beta-glucosidase in Gaucher fibroblasts by several mechanisms. Proc Natl Acad Sci USA. 2006;103(37):13813–8.
69. Amicus Therapeutics. Amicus therapeutics announces preliminary results of phase 2 study with Plicera(TM) for Gaucher disease 2009. http://ir.amicusrx.com/static-files/35813147-7c02-4311-b770-9279142ee4da
70. Narita A, Shirai K, Itamura S, Matsuda A, Ishihara A, Matsushita K, et al. Ambroxol chaperone therapy for neuronopathic Gaucher disease: a pilot study. Ann Clin Transl Neurol. 2016;3(3):200–15.
71. Istaiti M, Revel-Vilk S, Becker-Cohen M, Dinur T, Ramaswami U, Castillo-Garcia D, et al. Upgrading the evidence for the use of ambroxol in Gaucher disease and GBA related Parkinson: investigator initiated registry based on real life data. Am J Hematol. 2021;96(5):545–51.
72. Jiang W, Yi M, Maegawa GHB, Zhang H. Ambroxol improves skeletal and hematological manifestations on a child with Gaucher disease. J Hum Genet. 2020;65(3):345–9.
73. Fog-Tonnesen CK, Zago P, Malini E, Solanko LM, Peruzzo P, Bornaes C, et al. Arimoclomol as a potential therapy for neuronopathic Gaucher disease. bioRxiv. 2018:281824.
74. Aflaki E, Stubblefield BK, Maniwang E, Lopez G, Moaven N, Goldin E, et al. Macrophage models of Gaucher disease for evaluating disease pathogenesis and candidate drugs. Sci Transl Med. 2014;6(240):240ra73.
75. Aflaki E, Borger DK, Moaven N, Stubblefield BK, Rogers SA, Patnaik S, et al. A new glucocerebrosidase chaperone reduces α-synuclein and glycolipid levels in iPSC-derived dopaminergic neurons from patients with gaucher disease and parkinsonism. J Neurosci. 2016;36(28):7441–52.

76. Burbulla LF, Jeon S, Zheng J, Song P, Silverman RB, Krainc D. A modulator of wild-type glucocerebrosidase improves pathogenic phenotypes in dopaminergic neuronal models of Parkinson's disease. Sci Transl Med. 2019;11(514)
77. Cohen IJ, Kornreich L, Mekhmandarov S, Katz K, Zaizov R. Effective treatment of painful bone crises in type I Gaucher's disease with high dose prednisolone. Arch Dis Child. 1996;75(3):218–22.
78. Wenstrup RJ, Bailey L, Grabowski GA, Moskovitz J, Oestreich AE, Wu W, et al. Gaucher disease: alendronate disodium improves bone mineral density in adults receiving enzyme therapy. Blood. 2004;104(5):1253–7.
79. Bubbar V, Heras FL, Amato D, Pritzker KP, Gross AE. Total hip replacement in Gaucher's disease: effects of enzyme replacement therapy. J Bone Joint Surg Br. 2009;91(12):1623–7.
80. Hughes DAPG. Gaucher disease. In: Adam MP FJ, Mirzaa GM, et al, editor. GeneReviews® [Internet]. Seattle: University of Washington, Seattle; 2000 Jul 27 [Updated 2023 Dec 7].

7 Overview of Patients with Gaucher Disease from Iran

Daniel Zamanfar, Parastoo Rostami, and Noushin Rostampour

7.1 Abbreviations

ESR	Erythrocyte sedimentation rate
iPSC-dopaminergic	Induced pluripotent stem cell-dopaminergic
CHO cell	Chinese hamster ovary cell
DEXA	Dual-energy X-ray absorptiometry
Apo	Apolipoprotein
HDL	High-density lipoprotein
DNA	Deoxyribonucleic acid
NGS	Next-generation sequencing
X-ray	X-radiation
NKT	Natural killer

7.2 Introduction

This chapter reviews previous content by introducing several patients with GD, all from Iran and treated by pediatric endocrinologists in different cities. Patients presenting with different issues, like anemia, thrombocytopenia, liver enlargement, and bone pain, underwent several tests, including liver function test and bone marrow biopsies. They were ultimately diagnosed with GD through genetic testing. In contrast, some individuals were diagnosed with GD incidentally while being assessed for other health issues.

Introducing GD to other physicians and being aware of the symptoms of this disease will be effective in timely diagnosis and treatment and in preventing short- and long-term complications.

7.3 Patient 1

An 11-year-old girl, the first child of consanguineous parents and with a birth weight of 3100 g, was healthy until 6 months old. After that, her growth fell below the standard growth chart, leading to a diagnosis of failure to thrive (II) by a gastrologist.

Initial lab results indicated a platelet count of 140,000 per microliter and elevated tissue transglutaminase immunoglobulin A (TTG (IgA)) titer, confirming celiac disease through histologic findings. She began a gluten-free diet due to her failure to thrive. After 6 months with no improve-

D. Zamanfar
Thalassemia and Diabetes Research Center, Mazandaran University of Medical Sciences, Mazandaran, Iran

P. Rostami (✉)
Research Center for Growth and Development, Division of Endocrinology and Metabolism, Department of Pediatrics, Pediatrics Center of Excellence, Tehran University of Medical Sciences, Tehran, Iran

N. Rostampour
Metabolic Liver Disease Research Center, Isfahan University of Medical Sciences, Isfahan, Iran

© The Author(s), under exclusive license to Springer Nature Singapore Pte Ltd. 2025

P. Rostami, A. Talea (eds.), *Gaucher Disease*, https://doi.org/10.1007/978-981-96-4763-7_7

Table 7.1 Monitoring response to ERT over a year

	Treatment duration		
Parameters	Before ERT	5 months after ERT	12 months after ERT
Spleen diameter (mm)	126 × 50	112 × 37	Normal
WBC (μl)	4400	3700	5900
Hb (g/dl)	10.1	11.5	11.5
Platelet (μl)	99,000	135,000	160,000

Table 7.2 Monitoring response to ERT

	Treatment duration		
Parameters	Before ERT	20 months after ERT	26 months after ERT
Spleen diameter (mm)	156	120	Normal
Liver diameter (mm)	178	Normal	Normal
platelet (μl)	88,000	126,000	135,000

ment in growth, further evaluations showed decreased platelet counts compared to the earlier result.

Splenomegaly (127 × 43 mm) was found in her after 2 years, alongside a platelet count of 99,000 per microliter and reduced white blood cell count and level of hemoglobin. Due to persistent thrombocytopenia and pancytopenia, a bone marrow aspiration was performed, revealing the presence of Gaucher cells.

Whole exome sequencing identified the pathogenic variant c.[1226A > G]:[1448 T > C], p.[Asn 409ser]:[leu 488pro] in the *GBA1* gene, associated with GD1.

At 8 years and 5 months old, she received enzyme replacement therapy (ERT) with recombinant imiglucerase (Abcertin®, ISU Abxis, or Cerezyme®, Sanofi-Genzyme, whichever was available) at a dosage of 60 U/kg/biweekly. The course of response to ERT is shown in Table 7.1.

Learning Point

- This patient highlights the need to recognize celiac disease as a comorbidity-with GD and to suspect it in cases of inadequate weight gain despite ERT.
- GD should be considered in any patient with celiac disease who does not experience proper growth on a gluten-free diet, particularly if they also exhibit thrombocytopenia or splenomegal.

7.4 Patient 2

A 46-year-old male, born to consanguineous parents with a birth weight of 3150 grams, had no familial medical issues. At age 41, he presented with a 12 kg weight over 6 months, leading to the discovery of thrombocytopenia and, subsequently, splenomegaly during investigations. Bone marrow aspiration revealed Gaucher cells, confirming GD1 through the detection of the pathogenic homozygous variant c.[1060 G > A];[1060 G > A], (p.[Asp 354 Asn];[Asp 354 Asn]) in the *GBA1* gene via whole-exome sequencing.

At age 42, he began ERT with recombinant imiglucerase (Abcertin®, ISU Abxis, or Cerezyme®, Sanofi-Genzyme, whichever was available), at a dosage of 60 U/kg every 2 weeks. The course of the response to ERT for 26 months is shown in Table 7.2.

Learning Point

Consider Gaucher disease in unexplained weight loss at any age, particularly when associated with splenomegaly and thrombocytopenia.

7.5 Patient 3

A 6-year-and-4 month-old girl, born to nonconsanguineous parents with a birth weight of 2900 g, was admitted to the intensive unit care at 16 months due to sepsis. During her illness, she developed pancytopenia, which persisted despite improvement in sepsis. A bone marrow aspiration revealed the presence of Gaucher cells. A molecular study confirmed the pathogenic variant c.[1448 T > c];[1448 T > c];(p.[leu 483 pro];[leu leu 483 pro] in the *GBA1* gene.

ERT with recombinant imiglucerase (Abcertin®, ISU Abxis, or Cerezyme®, Sanofi-Genzyme, whichever was available) at 60 UI/kg/every 2 weeks was initiated. The response to ERT over 3 years is detailed in Table 7.3.

Learning Point
Numerous studies indicate that low beta-glucocerebrosidase activity is linked to impaired function of the immune system, potentially increasing the risk of infections before the onset of GD symptoms [1, 2].

7.6 Patient 4

A 22-year-old girl, born to a nonconsanguineous parent, had a history of primary hypothyroidism. Thrombocytopenia was revealed during follow-up for her condition. Further evaluation for persistent thrombocytopenia discovered splenomegaly on abdominal sonography, and bone marrow aspiration showed Gaucher cells.

B-glucocerebrosidase activity was 0.0%. Whole-exome sequencing revealed a pathogenic homozygous mutation, c. [1102 C > T]; [11.2 C > T], (p.[Arg 368 Cys]; [Arg 368 Cys]), in the *GBA1* gene.

ERT with recombinant imiglucerase (Abcertin®, ISU Abxis, or Cerezyme®, Sanofi-Genzyme, whichever was available) at a dosage of 30 U/kg every 2 weeks was initiated. The response to ERT over 2 years is mentioned in Table 7.4.

Learning Point
This patient had primary hypothyroidism as a comorbidity with GD, and due to the mild disease, ERT was initiated at a minimal dosage.

Table 7.3 Monitoring response to ERT

	Treatment duration			
Parameters	Before ERT	12 months after ERT	24 months after ERT	36 months after ERT
Spleen diameter (mm)	125 × 38	136 × 37	144 × 26	119 × 23
Liver diameter (mm)	77 × 35	108 × 55	98 × 46	86 × 33
WBC (μl)	4100	5400	6100	7900
Hb (g/dl)	9.9	11.1	11.6	13.3
Platelet (μl)	73,000	124,000	177,000	154,000

Table 7.4 Monitoring response to ERT

	Treatment duration		
Parameters	Before ERT	12 months after ERT	24 months after ERT
Spleen diameter (mm)	162 × 44	104 × 40	142 × 36
Liver diameter (mm)	161 × 52	137 × 48	Normal
Hb (g/dl)	11.6	11.6	11.4
Platelet (μl)	155,000	210,000	215,000

7.7 Patient 5

A 5-year-old girl, born to nonconsanguineous parents, was referred to a hematology clinic for splenomegaly without thrombocytopenia. Her parents had noticed gradual abdominal distention, and splenomegaly was confirmed through abdominal ultrasound. A bone marrow aspiration revealed Gaucher-like cells. B-glucocerebrosidase activity was 0.5 μmol/l/h (NL:>5). GD1 was confirmed by identifying a pathogenic homozygous mutation, c.[1448 T > C]; [1448 T > C], (p.[leu 483 pro]; [leu 483 pro]), in the *GBA1* gene.

At 14 months old, she received ERT with recombinant imiglucerase (Abcertin®, ISU Abxis, or Cerezyme®, Sanofi-Genzyme, whichever was available) at a dosage of 60 U/kg every 2 weeks. The response to ERT over a year is detailed in Table 7.5.

Learning Point
Given that splenomegaly is common in GD1, conducting genetic analysis or enzyme activity measurement prior to invasive procedures, like bone marrow aspiration or liver biopsy, is a sensible approach for diagnosis.

7.8 Patient 6

A 5-year-old boy, born to consanguineous parents, was referred to a hematology clinic for splenomegaly and anemia at 7 months old. At 6 months, he was evaluated for anemia; splenomegaly was detected during examination and later confirmed by ultrasound. A bone marrow aspiration at 8 months revealed histiocyte cells resembling Gaucher cells.

Beta-glucocerebrosidase activity was 0.5 mol/l/h (Nl > 5). Whole-exome sequencing identified a pathogenic homozygous variant, c.[1342G > C];[1342 G > C]; (p.[Asp 448 His];[Asp 448 His], in the *GBA1* gene.

Recombinant imiglucerase (Abcertin®, ISU Abxis, or Cerezyme®, Sanofi-Genzyme, whichever was available) at a dose of 60 U/kg every 2 weeks was initiated when he was 11 months old. At the age of 4 years, he exhibited abnormal eye movement, and an ophthalmology consultation diagnosed him with oculomotor apraxia. A brain MRI indicated susceptibility to GD2 or GD3, with a finding of mild parietal deep white matter changes and immature demyelination. The response to ERT after 1 year is detailed in Table 7.6.

Learning Point
Differentiating between GD1 and GD2 or GD3 relies on the later onset of neurologic symptoms despite existing genotype-phenotype correlations.

Table 7.5 Monitoring response to ERT

	Treatment duration	
Parameters	Before ERT	12 months after ERT
Spleen diameter (mm)	110 × 37	87 × 32
Liver diameter (mm)	164 × 48	100 × 46

Table 7.6 Monitoring response to ERT

	Treatment duration		
Parameters	Before ERT	24 months after ERT	36 months after ERT
Spleen diameter (mm)	70 × 33	79 × 40	88 × 35
Liver diameter (mm)	89 × 42	70 × 35	93 × 54
Hb (g/dl)	11.3	11.2	12

7.9 Patient 7

A 10-year-old boy, born to consanguineous parents, was referred to a hematology clinic at 8 months of age due to hepatosplenomegaly and anemia.

Beta-galactosidase enzyme activity was measured to evaluate for the possibility of Gaucher disease, yielding a result of 17.98 (*NL* = 200–2000 pmol/spot*20 h).

GD was confirmed by identifying a pathogenic homozygous variant, c.[1448 T > C]; [1448 T > C], (p.[leu 483 pro]; [leu 483 pro]), in the *GBA1* gene. At 7, he underwent splenectomy due to severe splenomegaly and abdominal discomfort despite ERT. At 7 years and 8 months, an X-ray for leg pain revealed an Erlenmeyer flask deformity in his left femur.

Recombinant imiglucerase (Abcertin®, ISU Abxis, or Cerezyme®, Sanofi-Genzyme, whichever was available) was initiated at 12 months old at a dosage of 60 U/kg every 2 weeks. His response to ERT over the first year is detailed in Table 7.7.

Learning Point
The patient had splenectomy due to significant splenomegaly and abdominal discomfort despite enzyme replacement therapy (ERT). The lack of response to ERT may be attributed to the use of different imiglucerase brands (Abcertin and Cerezyme) or autoantibody synthesis against imiglucerase. Therefore, using the same imiglucerase brand consistently and measuring autoantibodies in this condition is crucial.

7.10 Patient 8

The girl, aged 4 years and 10 months, was born to consanguineous parents. At 3 years old, she was referred to a gastroenterologist due to hepatosplenomegaly and thrombocytopenia. A liver biopsy indicated lysosomal storage disease, primarily suggesting Gaucher disease.

Testing revealed beta-glucocerebrosidase activity at less than 0.005 (*NL* = 0.06–0.2 U/mg protein).

A homozygous mutation, c.[1448 T > C]; [1448 T > C], (p.[leu 483 pro]; [leu 483 pro]), in the *GBA1* gene confirmed the diagnosis. At 3 years old, she began enzyme replacement therapy (ERT) with Abcertin® (ISU Abxis) or Cerezyme® (Sanofi-Genzyme) at a dosage of 60 U/kg every 2 weeks. Her response to ERT after 1 year is detailed in Table 7.8.

Learning Point
In a patient with hepatosplenomegaly and thrombocytopenia, Gaucher disease should be considered, and liver biopsy is not mandatory.

Table 7.7 Monitoring response to ERT

	Treatment duration	
Parameters	Before ERT	24 months after ERT
Spleen diameter (mm)	171 × 57	87 × 32
Liver diameter (mm)	106 × 46	86 × 33
Hb (g/dl)	10.3	12.6

Table 7.8 Monitoring response to ERT

	Treatment duration	
Parameters	Before ERT	12 months after ERT
Spleen diameter (mm)	130 × 55	92 × 37
Liver diameter (mm)	107 × 45	99 × 42
Platelet (μl)	109,000	155,000

Table 7.9 Monitoring response to ERT

	Treatment duration	
Parameters	Before ERT	12 months after ERT
Spleen diameter (mm)	112 × 45	108 × 37
Platelet (μl)	159,000	155,000

7.11 Patient 9

A 14-month-old boy from a consanguineous marriage was referred to a hematologist due to hepatosplenomegaly at 6 months. Bone marrow aspiration indicated a storage disease, with beta-glucocerebrosidase activity at 0.1 μmol/L/h (normal >1.5 μmol/L/h) and a homozygous variant, c.[1448 T > C]; [1448 T > C], (p.[leu 483 pro]; [leu 483 pro]), in the *GBA1* gene.

At 1 year old, he started enzyme replacement therapy (ERT) with Abcertin® (ISU Abxis) or Cerezyme® (Sanofi-Genzyme) at a dose of 60 U/kg every 2 weeks. His response to ERT over the 6-month period is detailed in Table 7.9.

> **Learning Point**
> The presence of hepatosplenomegaly in this patient, along with the absence of other malignancy risk factors, suggests Gaucher disease as the primary diagnosis, making bone marrow aspiration unnecessary.

7.12 Patient 10

A 5-year-old girl, born from a consanguineous marriage, was referred for splenomegaly without thrombocytopenia at 1 year and 6 months. Beta-glucocerebrosidase activity measured 2.8 (*NL* = 200–2000 pmol/spot*20 h). A homozygous variant, c.[1448 T > C]; [1448 T > C], (p.[leu 483 pro]; [leu 483 pro]), was identified in the *GBA1* gene. Enzyme replacement therapy (ERT) with Abcertin® (ISU Abxis) or Cerezyme® (Sanofi-Genzyme) was initiated at 1 year of age with a dosage of 60 U/kg every 2 weeks. Her ERT response after 6 months is detailed in Table 7.10.

> **Learning Point**
> Splenomegaly, with or without thrombocytopenia, is more indicative of Gaucher disease than hepatosplenomegaly.

7.13 Patient 11

A 16-year-10-month-old boy, born from a consanguineous marriage, was referred for splenomegaly with thrombocytopenia and anemia at 10. Bone marrow aspiration revealed Gaucher-like cells. Beta-glucocerebrosidase activity was low (1.3 nmol/ml/h, normal; 5-47). Molecular analysis indicated the variant compound heterozygous c.C12431(P.R 415c)-c.T1178c(p.L396p) in the *GBA*1 gene. Her parents did not agree to ERT at

Table 7.10 Monitoring response to ERT

Parameters	Treatment duration Before ERT	12 months after ERT
Spleen diameter (mm)	125 × 45	123 × 38
Platelet (μl)	Normal	Normal

Table 7.11 Monitoring response to ERT

Parameters	Treatment duration Before ERT	12 months after ERT	24 months after ERT	36 months after ERT
Spleen diameter (mm)	242 × 107	192 × 51	204 × 72	148 × 45
Liver diameter (mm)	151 × 52	117 × 35	112 × 41	131 × 38
Hb (g/dl)	7.3	9.7	12.1	14
Platelets (μl)	116,000	148,000	193,000	155,000

that time, but due to huge splenomegaly, progressive anemia, and thrombocytopenia, the patient underwent treatment with imiglucerase (Abcertin®) at a dosage of 60 U/kg every 2 weeks at 12. His ERT response for 36 months is detailed in Table 7.11.

Learning Point
Splenomegaly with hematologic abnormalities without malignancy risk factors is more indicative of Gaucher disease.

7.14 Patient 12

A 17-year-old boy, born from a nonconsanguineous marriage, was referred for splenomegaly and leg pain at 13. Bone marrow aspiration revealed storage cells. Beta-glucocerebrosidase activity was zero (5–47 nmol/ml/h). Molecular analysis detected the variant heterozygous c.[437C > T];[1226A > G, (p.[Ser146Leu];Asn409Leu]) in the *GBA1* gene.

ERT with recombinant imiglucerase (Abcertin®) at a dosage of 60 U/kg every 2 weeks was begun at 13. His ERT response for 48 months is detailed in Table 7.12.

Learning Point
Bone marrow aspiration is warranted in this patient due to leg pain, splenomegaly, and a suspicion of malignancy [3].

Table 7.13 summarizes all patients' information. The most common clinical manifestations and pathogenic variants are visceromegaly,

Table 7.12 Monitoring response to ERT

Parameters	Treatment duration Before ERT	12 months after ERT	24 months after ERT	36 months after ERT
Spleen diameter (mm)	140 × 83	146 × 64	144 × 66	102 × 35
Liver diameter (mm)	130 × 46	138 × 35	145 × 42	150 × 36
Hb (g/dl)	11	14.9	13.9	13.6
Platelets (μl)	120,000	235,000	274,000	235,000

hematological abnormalities, and c.[1448 T > C]; [1448 T > C], (p.[leu 483 pro]; [leu 483 pro]), respectively. Eight of our 12 patients were born to consanguineous parents, indicating an autosomal inheritance pattern of Gaucher disease. Neurological symptoms appeared in a patient with the pathogenic variant c.[1342G > C] (p.[Asp 448 His]), possibly linked to GD3, similar to another reported patient with the same variant (3). Patients 2, 4, 11, and 12, who exhibited no neurological symptoms until adulthood, may have GD1.

Table 7.13 Summary of all patients information

Patient no.	Sex	Age at diagnosis	Present symptom	Comorbidities	Consanguineous parent	Enzyme activity	Molecular analysis of the *GBA1* gene
1	Girl	6 months	Growth failure	Celiac disease	+	–	c.[1226A > G];[1448 T > C], p.[Asn 409ser];[leu 488pro]
2	Boy	46 years	Weight loss, splenomegaly, thrombocytopenia	–	+	–	c.[1060 G > A];[1060 G > A], (p.[Asp 354 Asn];[Asp 354 Asn])
3	Girl	6 years/4 months	Thrombocytopenia and sepsis	–	–	–	c.[1448 T > c];[1448 T > c];(p.[leu 483 pro];[leu leu 483 pro]
4	Girl	22 years	Thrombocytopenia	Primary hypothyroidism	–	0.0%	c.[1102 C > T]; [11.2 C > T], (p.[Arg 368 Cys]; [Arg 368 Cys])
5	Girl	5 years	Splenomegaly	–	–	[a]0.5 µmol/l/h	c.[1448 T > C]; [1448 T > C], (p.[leu 483 pro]; [leu 483 pro])
6	Boy	5 years	Splenomegaly and anemia	Progressive neurological symptoms	+	0.5 µmol/l/h	c.[1342G > C];[1342 G > C]; (p.[Asp 448 His];[Asp 448 His]
7	Boy	10 years	Hepatosplenomegaly and anemia	–	+	[b]17.98	c.[1448 T > C]; [1448 T > C], (p.[leu 483 pro]; [leu 483 pro])
8	Girl	4 years	Hepatosplenomegaly and thrombocytopenia	–	+	[c]0.005	c.[1448 T > C]; [1448 T > C], (p.[leu 483 pro]; [leu 483 pro])
9	Boy	14 months	Hepatosplenomegaly	–	+	0.1 µmol/L/h	c.[1448 T > C]; [1448 T > C], (p.[leu 483 pro]; [leu 483 pro])
10	Girl	5 years	Splenomegaly	–	+	[b]2.8	c.[1448 T > C]; [1448 T > C], (p.[leu 483 pro]; [leu 483 pro])
11	Boy	16 years/10 months	Splenomegaly and thrombocytopenia	–	+	[d]1.3	c.C12431(P.R 415c)-c.T1178c(p. L396p)
12	Boy	17 years	Splenomegaly and leg pain	–	–	[d]Zero	c.[437C > T];[1226A > G, (p.[Ser146Leu];Asn409Leu])

[a]Normal > 1.5 µmol/L/h
[b]Normal: 200–2000 pmol/spot 20 h
[c]Normal: 0.06–0.2 U/mg protein
dNormal: 5–47 nmol/ml/h

References

1. Liu J, Halene S, Yang M, Mistry PK. Gaucher disease gene GBA functions in immune regulation. Biol Sci. 2012;109(25):10018–23.
2. Zahran AM, Saad K, Elsayh KI, Abdou MAA, et al. Upregulation of Cytotoxic T-cells in pediatric patients with Gaucher disease. Sci Rep. 2022;12:4977.
3. Michelakakis H, Skardoutsou A, Mathioudakis J, Moraitou M, Dimitriou E, Voudris C, et al. Early-onset severe neurological involvement and D409H homozygosity in Gaucher disease: outcome of enzyme replacement therapy. Blood Cells Mol Dis. 2002;28(1):1–4.

MIX
Papier aus verantwortungsvollen Quellen
Paper from responsible sources
FSC® C105338

If you have any concerns about our products,
you can contact us on
ProductSafety@springernature.com

In case Publisher is established outside the EU,
the EU authorized representative is:
Springer Nature Customer Service Center GmbH
Europaplatz 3, 69115 Heidelberg, Germany

Printed by Libri Plureos GmbH
in Hamburg, Germany